Rheumatology: A Handbook for Community Nurses

JACKIE HILL MPhil, RGN, FRCN

Lecturer and Rheumatology Nurse Practitioner, Leeds

and

SARAH RYAN BSc, MSc, RGN

Clinical Nurse Specialist Rheumatology, Stoke on Trent

SERIES EDITOR

MARILYN EDWARDS

Specialist Practitioner, General Practice Nursing,
Bilbrook Medical Centre, Staffordshire

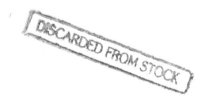
W

WHURR PUBLISHERS
LONDON AND PHILADELPHIA

© 2000 Whurr Publishers Ltd
First published 2000
by Whurr Publishers Ltd
19b Compton Terrace
London N1 2UN England and
325 Chestnut Street, Philadelphia PA 19106 USA

British Library Cataloguing-in-Publication Data
A catalogue record for this book is available from the British Library.

ISBN 1 86156 159 8

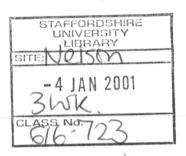
Printed and bound in Great Britain by Athenæum Press Ltd, Gateshead, Tyne & Wear.

Contents

Introduction

Arthritis and rheumatism are the most frequently self-reported long-standing conditions in the UK with an incidence of 80 per 1000 adult females and 40 per 1000 adult males (OPCS, 1989).

The majority of patients with rheumatic diseases are managed in the primary care setting. Musculoskeletal diseases and their associated problems account for 18.7% of all general practitioner (GP) consultations, although only about 4% of patients are referred to a hospital-based rheumatologist (Symmons and Bankhead, 1994). These are generally patients who have a disease such as rheumatoid arthritis (RA) or systemic lupus erythematosus (SLE) that is likely to affect the organs and systems in addition to the joints.

There is also evidence of an increased workload in the secondary sector reported by Kirwan (1996). He found that rheumatologists in the South West Regional Health Authority were engaging in more consultations, rising from 2663 in 1988 to 3485 in 1994. This represented a 19% increase in new patients and a 16% increase in follow-up consultations.

There is clearly an increased demand for rheumatology services in both care environments. The primary health care team is expected to ensure a seamless service between primary and secondary health care teams for these patients and in addition to provide the relevant expertise, support and advice. It is therefore essential that the staff concerned have the necessary knowledge and skills to provide a high quality service to this group of patients.

Innovative management of rheumatic disease, which has improved patient care within primary care, is examined in Chapter 1. The introduction of primary care groups, with its associated clinical governance, may result in rheumatology care having a higher profile in an ageing population. The benefits of shared care between the primary and secondary sectors can be experienced by most practices.

Because rheumatic conditions are so numerous, for the purposes of this book those most commonly seen in the community and those that are the most characteristic of their group are classified into five categories, which are discussed in Chapter 2. Information about other rheumatic diseases can be found in other texts (Hill, 1998a).

Many practice nurses are involved in the administration of injections or in monitoring drug therapy, often without appropriate training. Chapter 3 details the key issues involved in the common drug therapies, and provides useful reference data.

Most rheumatic diseases are chronic and debilitating. Patient education (PE) can improve the quality of life for many of these patients by empowering them and enabling them to take some control over their daily activities. Chapter 4 explains the benefits of PE and how the community nurse can assist the patient to cope with his/her condition.

Most diseases are managed most effectively by a multidisciplinary team. Appropriate management of rheumatic diseases requires the input of a range of health professionals, whose skills should be sought at diagnosis, not as a last resort. The role of each team member is discussed in Chapter 5. It should never be assumed, even if a patient has attended hospital, that the relevant services have been offered; they may not have been required at that time.

Psychological aspects of many diseases are often ignored, more through lack of knowledge than from design. Chapter 6 provides an insight into the variety of psychological issues pertinent to rheumatic diseases.

The final chapter lists the appropriate assessments that assist disease management. The Royal College of Nursing has provided guidelines for the administration of drugs; these should be followed to ensure safe practice. General information and useful addresses complete the chapter.

The book has been written in a question-and-answer format for ease of reference, with topics cross-referenced where appropriate. This handbook will enable readers to have the answers to common questions at their fingertips.

Chapter 1
Community Innovations in the Care of Rheumatic Diseases

The care of patients with rheumatic diseases has shifted from secondary to primary care over recent years. Although this increases the workload of the primary health care team, there are benefits for patients and carers, and increased educational opportunities for nurses. This chapter examines some of the innovations in community care for patients with rheumatic diseases.

Q1.1: How has health policy affected community care?

The 1989 Community Care Act (DoH, 1989) required assessment of the health care needs of the local community to be addressed through the planning and purchasing of appropriate services for patients. The social service department therefore took prime responsibility for the provision of social care, with the health authorities accountable for addressing health needs. The political ethos to involve those parties directly responsible for clinical care decisions led to many general practitioners (GPs) becoming fundholders and entering into contractual arrangements with providers of care, such as hospitals.

The end of the internal market and GP fundholding heralds yet another massive reorganization in the National Health Service (NHS) (Carnell, 1998). The political commitment to clinical governance provides the foundation for the current development of primary care groups (PCGs), which commenced commissioning of health care on 1 April 1999. PCGs are multidisciplinary and their

1

configuration is shown in Table 1.1, although there has been widespread variation as to how these groups have been configured and developed across the country (Willis, 1998).

Table 1.1 The constitution of PCGs

4–7	General practitioners
1–2	Community/practice nurses
1	Social services nominee
1	Lay member
1	Health authority representative
1	General officer

The Community Practitioner and Health Visitors Association supported a proposal to develop local nursing forums to provide their local PCG with the information necessary to provide appropriate care. The function of PCGs is shown in Table 1.2. Their overall objective is to develop primary care services that will improve the health of the community and reflect the principles of *The New NHS: Modern, Dependable* (DoH, 1998) shown in Table 1.3.

Table 1.2 Functions of PCGs

To identify health needs in the community

To improve the quality, equity and standards of care provided

To work closely with social services and other local government agencies to ensure coordination and integration of service delivery

To advise on, or commission directly, a range of hospital services for patients within their area to meet identified need

To integrate the delivery of primary and community health services

To work closely with the voluntary sector

To involve the public in the work of the groups

The British League Against Rheumatism (BLAR) is an organization comprising representatives from professional bodies and patient organizations. It has developed standards of care for patients with osteoarthritis (OA) and rheumatoid arthritis (RA), which are divided into two categories:

Table 1.3 Principles of the White Paper *The New NHS: Modern, Dependable*

A desire to modernize the NHS

An emphasis on health not just health services

A focus on the needs of individuals and communities

Collaboration between all agencies that can provide care

Source: DoH (1998).

- essential standards;
- desirable standards.

It is envisaged that these standards will become the benchmark to monitor the quality of care provided for these patients in both the primary and secondary health settings (BLAR, 1997). The standards relevant to primary care are shown in Q7.1 and Q7.2. PCG nurse board members have the opportunity to develop and improve standards of care for their PCG population.

Q1.2: What is shared care?

Shared care has been described as a joint participation between the GP and the hospital consultant in the planned delivery of care for patients with a chronic condition, including an enhanced information exchange over and above routine discharge and referral letters (Hickman et al., 1994). Barrett and Tones (1992) suggest that shared care involves an understanding of:

- each other's problems;
- the need for support;
- the need for training;
- the need for explicit written management protocols.

In certain chronic diseases, such as diabetes and asthma, shared management between the hospital and GP is well established. It is important to broaden this description to include other health professionals who are involved in the patient's care, including nurses, physiotherapists, occupational therapists, orthotists, pharmacists and chiropodists. Although patients will enter the hospital setting only for a defined purpose such as a day case, inpatient stay, outpatient review or occupational therapy provision, an effective relationship and communication strategy is required between all those professionals involved in the patient's care to ensure care delivery is effective and relevant for the intended recipient.

Drug Monitoring: An Example of the Potential for Shared Care Delivery

The British Society for Rheumatology (1992) recommended that all patients with RA be referred to a consultant rheumatologist, with the subsequent sharing of treatment between the hospital setting and general practice where appropriate. This is good clinical management, as early intervention in inflammatory conditions can reduce the likelihood of joint damage (Donnelly et al., 1992).

The consultant will assess the patient's clinical condition from the history, physical assessment and inflammatory parameters such as erythrocyte sedimentation rate (ESR), plasma viscosity (PV) and C-reactive protein (CRP). The findings from this encounter will determine whether the patient requires disease-modifying anti-rheumatic drugs (DMARDs) or cytotoxic agents to suppress disease activity (see Chapter 3).

Some hospital settings have a nurse specialist or practitioner who can comprehensively explain to the patient the purpose, administration and monitoring requirements of drug therapy. Each rheumatology unit is different and some patients will receive initial monitoring in the hospital setting, whilst others will require the GP to arrange this monitoring. Patients on DMARDs require regular blood tests and, depending on their medication, blood pressure or urinalyis. These investigations assist in the surveillance of the safety and efficacy of the medication.

It is important that a practitioner who has received the relevant education and training in this area reviews the results of such investigations. As it often falls into the domain of the practice nurse to share in the collective responsibility for the monitoring of such therapy, it is essential that the nurse is provided with all the relevant information, including:

- details about the patient's condition and the proposed treatment plan;
- information regarding the prescribed medication, e.g. dosage, side-effects, time of administration and any interactions;
- the safety parameters relating to blood, urinalysis and blood pressure measurements and the action to take if results fall outside the designated limits;
- the action to take if the patient experiences side-effects;
- a contact number to provide a quick, accessible means of communication to a knowledgeable practitioner familiar with the patient's care, should a problem arise.

Many rheumatology units recommend the use of a shared care booklet which contains information about the necessary blood tests and a contact number if the results fall below accepted parameters. Such a booklet can act as a good communication tool between different care settings and also enables the patient to become an active participant in his/her care delivery. Havelock (1998) found this method of communication worked well within both the primary and secondary health care setting. Her research revealed that the majority of patients were being adequately monitored with only 2% of the study population not receiving the intended monitoring regime.

A general practice of 2000 patients may have up to 140 diabetic patients but only 10–20 patients with RA, and only a small percentage of these will require DMARDs. It is therefore essential that the practice nurse receives the necessary education, training and support to carry out this practice effectively. Helliwell and O'Hara (1995) performed an audit of drug monitoring in the community, from which they proposed a number of recommendations (Table 1.4).

Q1.3: What are community clinics?

The philosophy governing the development of community clinics is the provision of a rheumatology care service within the patient's local environment. This may involve the consultant rheumatologist conducting a rheumatology clinic within a general practice surgery or local hospital. Potential advantages of this means of care provision include:

Table 1.4 Improving community drug monitoring

The development of general practice information packages containing patient information sheets, monitoring protocols, monitoring booklets, support services and contact points

Improvements in pathology laboratory collection services for GPs

A network of district nurses and/or community phlebotomists who are able to take blood from patients who are unable to go to the general practice surgery

Improved communication between the rheumatology department and the GP through the use of structured letters with clear guidance on prescriptions, monitoring and side-effects

---

Source: Adapted from Helliwell and O'Hara (1995).

- improving accessibility for the patient;
- regular consultant review for the patient;
- the consultant can develop working partnerships with community staff;
- increased educational opportunity for the GP.

Patients favour this method of care delivery primarily because they are reviewed in a familiar setting with a shorter waiting time and by the consultant each time (Goodwin, 1994). It has been reported that GP contact in clinics was infrequent, often because GPs were conducting their own general practice clinics at the same time and were unable to have an active role in the community clinic (Bailey et al., 1994; Helliwell, 1996). GPs acknowledge the need for postgraduate education in rheumatology and would welcome the opportunity to develop practical skills (Blaaw et al., 1995). It appears that unless time is specified for the GP to contribute to the community clinic then potential educational opportunities will be lost. The efficiency of community clinics has also been questioned as patients may still need to visit the hospital for certain investigations and the utilization of a consultant in the community is an expensive commodity (Snaith, 1994; Walker, 1994).

Q1.4: What preparation does the community health care team (CHCT) require?

If community care is to be a success then adequate time, resources and training must be made available to enable the CHCT to provide the full range of health care and support required for an effective patient-focused service (Arthritis Care, 1994).

Community nurses are engaged in an ever-expanding role. It is not possible to provide an effective service in the community until health professionals have received the necessary training and ongoing support to equip them to become involved in new care provision. Practice nurses regularly review patients on drug therapy and assess the efficacy of treatment, while district nurses or health visitors will see patients with RA or OA who have other health care problems. Patients will often use these encounters to seek advice about other aspects of their arthritis.

The hospital-based rheumatology service must provide educational opportunities for all community nurses and offer a flexible means of professional development. Evening or weekend educational sessions may be required. Dargie and Proctor (1998) refer to a disappointing 2% uptake at an educational project developed by the clinical nurse specialist designed to meet the needs of practice nurses. This suggests that the timing or cost of the project may have been prohibitive.

Some hospitals, including the Staffordshire Rheumatology Centre, are fortunate to have a hospital-based community rheumatology nurse. Her role involves visiting practice nurses and developing working relationships. She can respond to identified needs and spend time in one-to-one education or group sessions. This has involved educating practice nurses about the administration of intramuscular methotrexate and providing educational and reference material on aspects of rheumatological conditions. The facility of a helpline service, which all community health workers can utilize, provides a mechanism whereby the hospital can be contacted to provide advice on clinical situations.

Q1.5: What are the outcomes of community-based educational programmes?

Community-based educational programmes have been shown to be effective in encouraging people with arthritis to adopt self-management techniques to cope with their arthritis (Barlow et al., 1996) and these are discussed in Chapter 4. Participants with OA or RA reported benefit in terms of their perceived ability to manage their arthritis, increased use of self-management strategies such as exercise, improved psychological well-being and a reduction in patient visits to the GP. Similar programmes can be held in general practice surgeries and would usually involve input from both the secondary and primary care team.

It is important to encourage the development of community-based programmes, as the care of patients with OA is often managed entirely in the community. OA is a chronic condition that can affect physical, psychological and social well-being (see Chapter 2). These patients require education to enable them to learn more about their arthritis and to gain the knowledge and confidence to undertake self-care.

One example of good practice is the Haywood Hospital, Staffordshire Rheumatology Centre, where an arthritis care group holds an evening exercise session in the hydrotherapy pool to enable people to continue with their exercises and enjoy social contact. Such innovations are necessary to enable patients to take an active role in the management of their condition.

Q1.6: What are nurse-led clinics?

Over the last decade there has been a major development with nurses expanding their skills and conducting nurse-led clinics in clinical areas including diabetes, asthma and rheumatology. These clinics allow partnership, intimacy and reciprocity to evolve between the nurse and the patient. The nurse's role grows from a supportive into a therapeutic one. Instead of concentrating exclusively on preventing deterioration, the nurse seeks to promote adaptation to the effects of the condition, which is an essential component for patients living with a chronic illness. Key nursing functions stated by Wilson-Barnett in 1984 provide the philosophy for nurse-led clinics that is still relevant today, including:

- understanding illness and treatment from the patient's viewpoint;
- providing continuous psychological care during illness and critical events;
- helping people cope with illness or potential health problems;
- providing comfort;
- coordinating treatment and other events affecting the patient.

Phelan et al. (1992) surveyed the roles of rheumatology nurse specialists and found that the majority perceived the counselling and education of patients to be the pivotal feature of their role. Mooney (1996) is a hospital-based rheumatology nurse practitioner who conducts clinics for patients with arthritis in general practice surgeries. Benefits of this care provision include:

- increased patient satisfaction;
- increased opportunity for patient education including the involvement of the multidisciplinary team;
- the provision of ongoing support;
- the opportunity to discuss any problems with a knowledgeable practitioner;
- continuity of care as patients are reviewed by the same nurse at each visit;
- a focus on prevention rather than crisis management.

The nurse is also able to provide specialist advice to the GP. Hill et al. (1994) reported that patients attending a nurse-led clinic reported less pain, less anxiety, increased knowledge and satisfaction when compared with their counterparts attending a consultant-led clinic.

Dargie and Proctor (1993) developed a community-based arthritis clinic within their own general practice surgery. This clinic achieved its objectives of providing an easily accessible service for the assessment, support, education and monitoring of patients and their families. The clinics were able to tailor services to meet individual needs and enabled patients to take an active role in care management so that they could cope with the condition on a daily basis.

Conclusion

It is clearly recognized that the numbers of patients treated within the community setting will continue to grow. This is the objective of health policy and is evident in pre-registration nurse preparation. A structured framework must exist to address training, communication and care guidelines between all sectors involved in care provision to ensure that the patient receives a care system that matches identified need.

Chapter 2
The Rheumatic Diseases

The term 'rheumatic diseases' describes over 200 conditions that affect the joints, bones, muscles and soft tissues of the musculoskeletal system. Their severity ranges from mild, self-limiting problems to severe, life-threatening illnesses. They occur in all age-groups including children and babies but their prevalence increases with age. The problem is enormous, with one person in seven in the UK affected by a significant rheumatic disease and over three million adults physically disabled by their effects (Martin et al., 1988). Approximately 20% of the population experience painful joints and 13% suffer from painful feet in any given month (Blaxter, 1990) (see Table 2.1).

In an ageing population, the number of people affected by a rheumatic disease is inevitably increasing. The most common rheumatic diseases seen in the community are classified into five categories (Table 2.2).

Table 2.1 Prevalence of common rheumatic symptoms

| Symptom | Sex | Prevalence (%) Age band | | | |
		18–44	45–64	65+	All ages
Painful joints	Male	12.2%	26.9%	50.5%	20.0%
	Female	10.9%	33.3%	44.7%	23.9%
Painful feet	Male	10.1%	14.6%	17.4%	12.9%
	Female	10.3%	21.3%	27.9%	16.9%

Source: Blaxter (1990).

Table 2.2 Common rheumatic diseases

Category	Disease
Joint failure	Osteoarthritis (OA)
Inflammatory joint disease	Rheumatoid arthritis (RA)
	Ankylosing spondylitis
	Gout
	Psoriatic arthritis
Bone diseases	Osteoporosis
Connective tissue disorders	Systemic lupus erythematosus (SLE)
	Scleroderma
Non-articular conditions	Back pain
	Soft tissue rheumatism

Osteoarthritis (OA)

The osteoarthritic disorders are a heterogeneous group of conditions affecting the synovial joints. They are found throughout the world and are the most common form of rheumatic disease in the UK. There was a 2% increase in incidence between 1981 and 1991 (Charlton et al., 1995). They are major source of distress to the patient and a significant health care problem for society as a whole. A practice of 10 000 patients will probably include 3000 with OA, although many will not consult their general practitioner (GP) about it (Bird, 1993).

OA becomes increasingly common with age and there is no known aetiology or cure. However, the nurse can play an important role in ensuring that the patient remains as pain free, active and independent as possible.

Q2.1: What are the pathological features of OA?

The characteristics of OA are:

- damage to the articular cartilage;
- increased activity in the subchondral bone;
- marginal osteophyte formation.

In the early stages, the articular cartilage (the surface of the bone) thins and, over time, the underlying bone thickens and broadens as if to reduce the load on the articular cartilage. This broadening is the formation of osteophytes (sometimes referred to as 'lipping' as they resemble lips when seen on X-ray) produced by the growth of fibro-cartilage and bone at the joint margins. As the disease worsens, the loss of further cartilage leads to joint-space narrowing. In advanced cases, there is moderate patchy synovitis (inflammation of the synovium), the synovial membrane and joint capsule thicken and increased amounts of synovial fluid are produced. Sclerosis and cysts also occur in the subchondral bone (Figure 2.1).

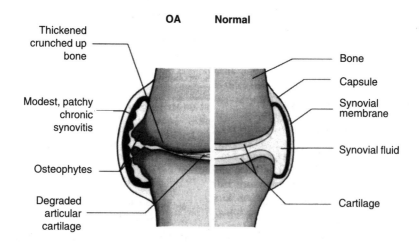

Figure 2.1 OA versus normal joint.
Reproduced with kind permission of Geoff Hill.

Q2.2: What is the difference between primary and secondary OA?

No predisposing cause can be identified in primary OA. It is termed 'generalized osteoarthritis' (GOA) when a number of joints are involved. GOA is more commonly found in women than men, particularly following the menopause. Characteristically, it involves the distal interphalangeal joints of the hands, which become swollen and painful. The pain eventually subsides, leaving nodules at the joint margins called Heberden's nodes (Figure 2.2). There is usually simultaneous involvement of other joints, typically the knees and hips.

In secondary OA there is a predisposing cause such as joint trauma, anatomical abnormality or metabolic disorder. Males and females are affected equally and normally a single joint or small number of joints is involved.

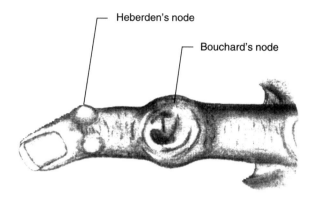

Figure 2.2 Heberden's and Bouchard's nodes.
Reproduced with kind permission of Geoff Hill.

Q2.3: Who is affected by OA?

OA affects more women than men. Below age 45, it is slightly more common in men, but it is more common in older women, coinciding with the age of the menopause. Peak onset is between ages 50 and 60 (Arthur, 1998). X-ray evidence shows that most people are affected by age 65, with over 80% affected by age 75 (Cooper, 1998). Fortunately, radiological evidence does not necessarily indicate that the disease is symptomatic, and it is those that display symptoms who require treatment.

Q2.4: Which are the most commonly affected sites?

OA can affect any synovial joint, but the most common sites are:

* hips;
* knees;
* distal interphalangeal joints (fingertip joints);
* first carpometacarpal joint (base of the thumb);
* apophyseal joints of the spine;
* first metatarsophalangeal joint (hallux valgus).

Most commonly affected are the joints necessary for an upright posture and prehensile grip. This has led some rheumatologists to postulate that these joints have not evolved sufficiently to undertake their present duty (Dieppe, 1995).

Q2.5: How does OA develop?

OA usually develops gradually over several years. At first, many people hardly notice their symptoms apart from the occasional aches and pains of ageing, usually associated with use of a particular joint. In these people the disease never really becomes a burden and life proceeds at a slower but acceptable pace. However, in some patients the disease begins to affect their lives in profound ways. It starts with mild stiffness of the joint and aching of nearby muscles that gradually increase in severity. Patients notice greater difficulty getting out of bed or climbing stairs as a result of pain, stiffness or decreasing range of movement. Occasionally, patients present with sudden onset of pain following joint trauma such as a fall. The symptoms do not subside, but worsen over a couple of weeks. Here it is probable that there was an existing underlying asymptomatic OA, which the trauma has aggravated into full-blown disease.

Q2.6: Are there any risk factors for OA?

There are a number of factors that predispose humans to OA, which are discussed individually below. The site and severity of the disease are determined by factors such as joint trauma and abnormalities, occupational and leisure activities (Figure 2.3).

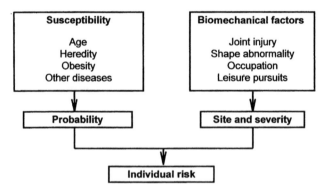

Figure 2.3 Factors contributing to the individual risk of OA.

The Effect of Ageing (see Q2.3)

The incidence of hand, hip and knee disease increases with age (Oliveria et al., 1995). However, by the eighth decade the incidence levels off in all three sites in both sexes (Figure 2.4).

Hand

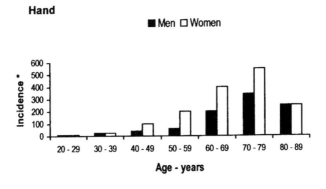

Knee

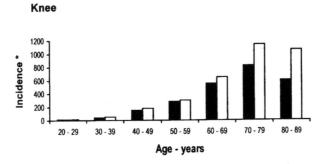

Hip

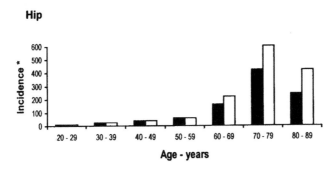

* Incidence is per 100,000 per year

Figure 2.4 Incidence of OA of the hand, knee and hip.
Source: Data from the Fallon Community Health Plan.

Obesity

OA of the knee is more common in overweight patients and if the patient is obese, it is more likely be bilateral rather than unilateral (Davis et al., 1991). It is also about twice as common in women as men. Excessive weight does not appear to be a risk factor in all forms of OA. There is little evidence that it is implicated in OA of the hip, although this is a weight-bearing site.

It has long been speculated that patients become overweight because their disease degenerates, causing immobility and difficulty with exercise. However recent evidence from the United States indicates the opposite. The body mass index of patients measured between 1948 and 1951 was shown to be a predictor of radiographic knee OA some 36 years later (Davis et al., 1991). This finding shows that obesity can cause OA rather than be the result of it. Research also suggests that weight loss reduces the risk of OA of the knee (Felson et al., 1992). This finding has exciting implications for nurses working in primary care, where the majority of patients and potential patients are managed. Weight-reduction educational programmes, instigated by nurses, could play a significant part in the prevention of OA of the knee, increase the general well-being of individual patients and contribute to the financial health of the country.

Genetic Influences

In certain types of OA, there is evidence of a strong genetic component, mainly in women. The most common inherited form of the disease is primary GOA, first described by Kellgren and Moore (1952) in which the patient exhibits:

- Heberden's nodes (Figure 2.2, p. 13);
- Bouchard's nodes (Figure 2.2);
- premature degeneration of articular cartilage in many joints.

Other Diseases

There are a number of diseases that are associated with OA, including diabetes mellitus, hypertension and hyperuricaemia (Cooper, 1998).

Biomechanical Factors

Mechanical risk factors in OA are trauma and joint loading.

(a) Trauma. The joint can be traumatized in two ways:

(1) Previous unintentional injury. Fractures appear to predispose humans to develop OA. The most commonly affected sites are:

- femoral shaft   leading to OA of the hip;
- humerus   leading to OA of the shoulder;
- scaphoid   leading to OA of the wrist;
- tibia   leading to OA of the ankle.

Many young men who sustain injuries such as cruciate ligament damage or meniscal tears, playing contact sports such as rugby and football, frequently develop OA of the knee later in life.

(2) Previous surgery. The most notable culprit is meniscectomy. Most studies undertaken have reported an increased frequency of subsequent OA (Cooper et al., 1994).

(b) Joint loading and stress. Joints have evolved to be efficient load-bearing structures. However, if the joint shape is abnormal it can lead to excessive stresses in areas that are incapable of withstanding them. Some childhood hip disorders such as slipped femoral epiphysis, Perthes' disease and congenital dislocation of the hip are known to result in OA, which has usually developed by the age of 35 or earlier.

Occupation

As repetitive use of specific groups of joints appears to increase the risk of OA in particular individuals, occupation must be considered a relevant factor. For instance OA of the hip is common amongst farmers (Croft et al., 1992), and more common in manual workers than those with sedentary jobs (Cooper, 1995). Activities that combine kneeling or squatting with high physical demands are associated with OA of the knee.

Leisure Activities

Sporting activities that involve repetitive use of weight-bearing joints, such as athletics or football, do not appear to increase the risk of OA. It is only when the joint sustains injury that leisure activities lead to increased risk.

Q2.7: What are the signs and symptoms of OA? (See Q2.5)

The most frequent early symptoms of OA are intermittent diffuse aches or pains, usually when the joint is used. Mild stiffness and a reduction in the range of movement can also ensue. However, of all symptoms (Table 2.3) pain is the most feared and frequently reported. It is usually brought on by use of the affected joint and is often accompanied by tenderness around the joint margins. Almost all patients experience use pain, but only 50% report pain at rest and 30% nocturnal pain. Pain can also influence psychological factors such as anxiety and depression. Total pain appears to correlate with anxiety, whilst depression is related to pain severity (Summers et al., 1988).

Table 2.3 Signs and symptoms of OA

Signs:
Tender spots around the joint margin
Swelling of the area around the affected joint
Crepitus (cracking of the joint)
Signs of mild inflammation
Joint effusion
Instability
Reduced range of movement

Symptoms:
Pain related to movement (may be present at rest)
Stiffness and gelling of the joint (relieved by movement)
Joint feels tight
Loss of the full range of movement
Joint feels unstable
Functional limitations

Q2.8: How is OA managed?

The British League Against Rheumatism (BLAR) has published nationally agreed standards of care for people with OA and RA. They provide a benchmark for quality in both primary and secondary care and can be used as an audit tool and to provide guidance, which should lead to equity of care for patients.

At present OA is incurable and so the aims of management must be to:

- relieve the symptoms;
- minimize the risk of onset or progression;
- optimize function;
- improve the quality of the patient's life.

To achieve these goals it may be necessary to use several therapeutic modalities (Table 2.4) employing the skills of a multidisciplinary team of health care professionals. However, it is only if drug therapy or surgery is used that significant involvement of the medical profession is needed and this has been acknowledged by GPs themselves (Bird, 1994). Nurses are increasingly acknowledged as central figures in the care of people with rheumatic diseases, and nurse-led clinics have been introduced in outpatient departments (Hill, 1985; Ryan, 1995a) and primary care (Dargie and Proctor, 1993, 1994). Nursing intervention can be based on the Royal College of Nursing (RCN) Rheumatology

Table 2.4 Therapeutic interventions for OA

Intervention	Effect
Patient education	Empowerment, increased self-efficacy, knowledge, coping skills, self-management skills, symptom relief
Physiotherapy General exercise Hydrotherapy	Increased range of motion, increase muscle bulk, reduction of pain, increased sense of well-being
Footwear, orthoses, aids and appliances	Pain relief, reduction of impact loading, reduction of joint stress, independence, security of unstable joints
Relaxation techniques	Reduction of anxiety, reduction in pain perception
Dietary advice	Weight reduction, reduction of joint stress, prevention of joint stress
Complementary therapy	Pain relief, reduction in anxiety, feeling of well being
Local and systemic drug therapy	Symptom relief
Surgery	Pain relief

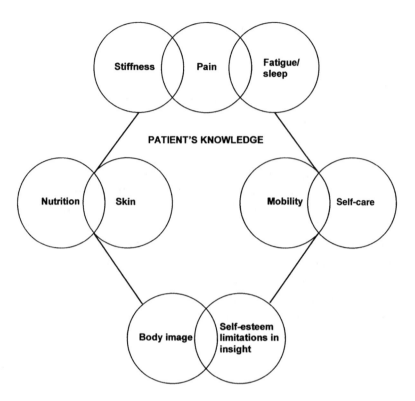

Figure 2.5 The RCN Rheumatology Nursing Forum Problem Model.
Reproduced with kind permission of the RCN.

Nursing Forum Problem Model (Figure 2.5) which incorporates all aspects of patient care including potential psychosocial problems.

Q2.9: What is patient education (PE)?

PE plays a pivotal role in the management of OA, not merely as a method of imparting information, but as a means of enabling the patient to become an active participant rather than a recipient of care. Patients and carers are encouraged to take control of the management of their disease and this has proved to be an effective strategy (Hampson et al., 1993). The PE programme for those with OA should include an assessment of their perception of the disease and how it limits their life. An explanation should be included of the disease process, pain control, available treatments, the role of diet, coping strategies, communication and self-help. PE is discussed in detail in Chapter 4.

Q2.10: Does physiotherapy help?

One of the 'essential standards' laid down in the BLAR document is an explanation of the role of exercise as a possible treatment for OA. Not all patients will need to see a physiotherapist. For elderly patients with mild OA, a general exercise regime or regular swimming sessions will improve their general fitness, reduce levels of pain and increase feelings of well-being. Daily quadriceps exercises are particularly important for those with OA of the knee.

There are many forms of exercise but low-impact aerobics (Minor, 1994) and fitness walking (Kovar et al., 1992) decrease levels of pain and improve disability in patients with OA of weight-bearing joints (see Q5.7 and 5.8). Patients with moderate to severe disease will require more specific expert help, which may include ultrasound (Q5.14) or hydrotherapy (Q5.17).

Q2.11: How important are footwear, walking aids, orthoses and appliances? (See also Chapter 5)

Footwear

The importance of footwear cannot be overrated in OA of the lower limb. Surgical shoes are not always indicated and frequently off-the-shelf trainers are ideal. They are designed to absorb impact during walking, so reducing pain and improving mobility. Some trainers have suitable insoles but others may require specially tailored inserts (see Q5.26).

Walking Aids

The purpose of a walking aid is to reduce stress on the affected limb. A simple walking stick can reduce pain, increase mobility and provide an additional sense of security to the patient. A walking stick should always be measured for the individual (see Q5.19), and must be held in the hand opposite to the affected leg. If both legs are affected, a walking frame will be more appropriate.

Unfortunately, many patients regard walking aids as a sign that they are 'crippled' or are 'giving in'. These patients may need to be counselled. Le Gallez (1990) suggests that altering their perception of the aid can persuade some patients to use it. Useful ploys are to liken the aid to a painkiller or to stress that it need not be used continually.

Orthoses

People with OA have reduced proprioception: the awareness, without looking, of the position of parts of the body in space. This contributes to the feeling of instability, which is often described by patients with OA of the knees, that their knees 'will let them down' (Marks et al., 1993). Elasticated bandages and tubigrip-type support can help these patients. For those with clinically unstable joints a brace can decrease pain, improve function and provide a feeling of security.

Pain is often a persistent problem when OA affects the carpometacarpal joint at the thumb base. This apparently small problem can become very disabling because it affects the pinch grip necessary for so many daily functions. A small splint can often help to reduce pain and stabilize the joint.

Aids and Appliances

OA can cause major functional problems and considerable levels of disability. Washing, dressing and preparing meals can be made difficult by hand problems. Holding a pen or using a keyboard can be troublesome for clerical workers. As well as the obvious problems of ambulation, OA of the lower limb can create problems getting in and out of bed or a chair, while getting off the toilet can become a major event and using a bath can be impossible. A visit to or by an occupational therapist will pay dividends in these cases (see Q5.20).

> **Q2.12: Do relaxation techniques, dietary advice and complementary therapy help?**

All these therapies can have a place in the treatment of OA. Relaxation can help patients to control their pain. Maintaining a reasonable weight is both preventive and therapeutic. Complementary therapies include the use of transcutaneous nerve stimulation (TENS units), useful for single rather than multiple joint pain relief, and acupuncture helps some patients (see Q5.15, 5.16).

Q2.13: Which drug-delivery systems are used?

Oral

The majority of patients who develop symptomatic OA require some form of drug therapy but when drugs are used the emphasis must be on safety. Many OA patients are elderly with impaired renal or hepatic function. These patients may also be taking drugs for other illnesses and drug interactions must be anticipated. Non-steroidal anti-inflammatory drugs (NSAIDs) are prescribed by 77% of GPs as the principal treatment in OA. However, NSAIDs increase the risk of gastrointestinal (GI) complications and predispose to GI bleeds; 80% of deaths from GI bleeds are in patients who have recently taken NSAIDs. Consequently, before using an NSAID it is good practice to try alternatives. Many patients cope well on paracetamol 1 g four times daily. Codeine, by itself or in combination, or dextropropoxyphene is also used successfully. If the desired therapeutic effect is not achieved, an NSAID can also be used. Ibuprofen appears to produce fewer, less serious side-effects than many NSAIDs and can be given at doses up to 600 mg three times daily. This should be tried for at least three weeks before moving to a more potent NSAID. All NSAIDs should be taken with or after food to minimize GI side-effects. Further information is given in Chapter 3.

Local

Pain can be relieved by applying heat or ice to the affected area and a patient information sheet on pain relief is shown in Chapter 4 (Figure 4.3). Many patients find heat helpful and preparations such as Deep Heat® can be bought over the counter. NSAID creams and gels are efficient at reducing pain in the hands and knees and are relatively safe compared with NSAID tablets.

Capsaicin cream, made from capsicum (pepper plant), reduces substance P locally. This substance is an excitatory neurone transmitter released by sensory neurones, which when inhibited reduce pain transmission. It is applied two to four times daily but patients should be warned that it often causes a burning sensation on the first few applications, although this reduces with regular use.

Intra-articular (IA) Injections

IA injections place drugs directly into the joint space or into soft tissue, giving a short-term reduction in symptoms. If a knee effusion is present, it is usually aspirated before the drug is instilled. This aids mobility and decreases the patient's discomfort.

Corticosteroids: A local injection of corticosteroid can be a very effective method of reducing pain, particularly when used on inflamed knees or at the thumb base.

Hyaluronate: A number of proprietary preparations of hyaluronate are available. They are given by IA injection for OA of the knees, usually five to six injections at weekly intervals. Those with more severe OA are likely to get the best response and, apart from occasional local reactions, there are few side-effects.

Q2.14: When is surgery used?

In advanced cases, where conservative treatments have failed, surgery may be an option. It is used predominantly for pain relief rather than to return normal function. The most pressing case is severe, unremitting nocturnal or rest pain that interrupts sleep regularly. The most successful procedures are hip replacement, followed by knee replacement (Sturdy, 1998a). These can transform the lives of patients but it should be made clear that arthroplasties have a finite life that depends on the patient's lifestyle, weight and age. Revision surgery is becoming more common but appears to be less satisfactory than the original.

Q2.15: How important is psychosocial support?

Psychosocial support can be very important for someone in pain and with diminished function. Patients with jobs may experience problems in the workplace that require a workplace visit or a consultation with the Disablement Resettlement Officer. Family support is essential, particularly if tasks of daily living, such as shopping, become difficult and a Disabled Parking Permit can enable patients to feel more in control of their everyday life. Social services can give advice on financial help and home alterations that may become necessary.

Voluntary organizations such as Arthritis Care and the Arthritis Research Campaign provide much assistance and local support groups exist in many areas of the country.

Case Study

Jane is a 68-year-old married woman with a seven-year history of pain in her knees. Her GP diagnosed primary OA three years ago. She was relatively well controlled on paracetamol 1 g four times daily for the first few years but as the pain became worse she was changed to co-proxamol to a maximum of eight tablets a day. About 18 months ago her pain increased and she was prescribed ibuprofen 600 mg three times daily.

Increasing pain and disability encouraged her to make an appointment at the nurse-led arthritis clinic at her health centre. She was interviewed and assessed on her:

- *knowledge of her disease and treatment options;*
- *pain;*
- *functional ability;*
- *social circumstances.*

On examination she was somewhat obese and her knees were tender to touch. She had hypertension controlled by drug therapy, but was otherwise fit and healthy. Her first priority was to reduce weight and she was referred to the dietitian. She was advised to wear trainers with soft inserts to reduce the stress on her knees when walking. Jane was told that she could supplement her NSAID with paracetamol (maximum eight daily) when necessary and she was taught how to apply heat or cold to her joints. Jane was reviewed monthly. Her PE programme included a home exercise programme, pain control methods and coping strategies.

Jane progressed well for a further nine months, when her right knee flared up and started to cause nocturnal pain which restricted her sleep. The knee felt unstable and Jane's function deteriorated, restricting her ability to shop and perform household tasks, making her feel depressed and anxious for the future.

An X-ray showed severe OA of the right knee, whilst the left knee remained stable. She was referred to the local hospital for a surgical opinion which resulted in a placement on the waiting list for a total knee replacement. Palliative treatment from the health centre comprised IA steroid injections, provision of a knee support and a walking stick. She was encouraged to carry out muscle-strengthening exercises at home, and to apply topical NSAID gels to her right knee. Because she encountered problems getting in and out of the bath a bath board and hand grip were installed, and a raised toilet seat fitted.

After several months a total knee replacement was undertaken which left Jane almost pain free, very soon after the surgery. A home assessment was made and physiotherapy arranged and she was discharged to the care of her husband and the district nurse. Jane attended the physiotherapy department at the hospital until she gained an appropriate range of movement and was eventually discharged from the hospital.

Her left knee still causes her pain, particularly because she is far more active than previously, but the education she has received from the nursing clinic has held her in good stead. She also knows that she can always return to clinic or phone the helpline for further assistance.

Some Common Questions

Q2.16: Are there any blood tests for OA?

No, there are no tests that will help the diagnosis. However, patients on NSAIDs may experience gastric oozing and become anaemic and this can be identified by full blood count.

Q2.17: What tests aid diagnosis?

The principal diagnostic test is a straight X-ray. This will confirm the diagnosis but severity on X-ray does not always mean the patient will suffer severe pain or disability. Blood tests, such as for rheumatoid factor, can help to eliminate other forms of arthritis.

Q2.18: Do special diets help?

There is at present no research to confirm that any particular food, additive or vitamin has either positive or detrimental effects on OA. The best diet is a well-balanced diet and those who are overweight will need to reduce weight.

Q2.19: How much exercise is recommended?

General exercise is not detrimental in OA, but patients should pace their activities, resting between periods of exercise (see Q5.24). Vigorous tasks are best undertaken in the morning, and it is better to avoid activities that cause severe pain. It can be helpful to take a couple of analgesics as a prophylactic measure before an activity that the patient knows causes him/her pain. Patients with OA often experience inactivity stiffness after sitting for long periods so it is better for them to get up and walk around frequently. Perhaps the best recommendation for exercise and rest is 'little and often'.

Q2.20: Does OA affect sexual activity?

Sexual intercourse can be problematic, particularly when pain in the hips or knees causes abduction problems. It is possible to discuss this quite openly with patients during the course of routine procedures such as taking cervical smears. Advice regarding positioning and prophylactic drug therapy can help to overcome the problem.

Q.2.21: Do patients pass OA on to their children?

Children of patients with GOA have an increased chance of developing this disease in middle age; daughters have a 50% chance of inheriting it from their mothers. The risk of inheriting knee OA is smaller. However, in the interests of good preventive medicine, nurses should encourage children, particularly daughters, of those with GOA or OA of the knee to exercise regularly and avoid becoming overweight.

Q2.22: Do drugs cure OA?

No, drugs can only alleviate the symptoms.

Q2.23: Should analgesics be taken on a regular basis?

Analgesics can be taken in two ways, either 'on demand' or 'regularly'. In general, on demand analgesics should be taken when the patient knows an activity is going to cause pain or the pain is particularly bad. Regular ingestion is used to suppress unremitting pain.

Q2.24: Are oral steroids of use?

There is no justification for the use of oral steroids in the treatment of OA at present.

Q2.25: Does the weather affect OA?

The weather may temporarily affect symptoms of OA such as pain and stiffness, but it does not cause OA or have any effect on the underlying disease.

Rheumatoid Arthritis (RA)

Rheumatoid arthritis was the name used to describe an 'inflammatory affection of the joints' by Sir Archibald Garrod in 1859. It is a chronic, inflammatory systemic condition and although it affects all age-groups it rarely occurs before puberty. At present RA is incurable but new drug therapies and earlier aggressive treatment can lessen the impact of the disease and any ensuing disability. The nurse can play a pivotal therapeutic role in caring for patients, ensuring they are educated and empowered, which will enable them to take control of their illness and their lives.

Q2.26: What are the pathological features of RA?

RA is characterized by an immune-driven chronic inflammation affecting the synovial membrane, which lines joint capsules and tendon sheaths of the body. The pathological changes usually occur in three stages (Matthew and Humphreys, 1994):

(1) cellular;
(2) inflammatory;
(3) destructive.

Cellular Stage

Initially the synovial membrane is affected and the joints become warm, swollen and tender causing some restriction of movement. Lymphocytes and plasma cells aggregate forming lymphoid follicles, which synthesize and secrete rheumatoid factors. These in turn react with immunoglobulins to form immune complexes.

Inflammatory Stage

Activation of the complement system leads to large numbers of granulocytes accumulating in the synovial fluid. Destruction of granulocytes during the inflammatory process results in the release of lysosomal enzymes.

Destructive Stage

The primary target for destruction is the articular hyaline cartilage. Vascular granulation tissue called 'pannus' produces proteases and collagenases that erode demineralized bone and cartilage. The pannus erodes the cartilage from the outer margins.

Abnormal joint stress is also produced by:

- unremitting synovitis;
- large-joint effusions;
- osteoporotic changes.

The combination of all these factors can lead to the joint instability, subluxation and deformity that are characteristic of RA (Figure 2.6).

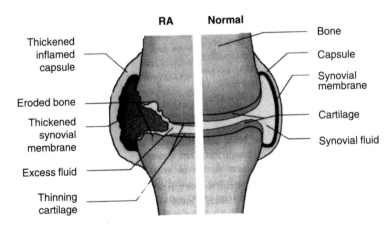

Figure 2.6 RA versus normal joint.
Reproduced with kind permission of Geoff Hill.

Q2.27: How is RA classified?

The currently accepted scheme for classifying RA was produced by the American Rheumatism Association (ARA; Arnett et al., 1988) (see Table 2.5). At least four criteria must be fulfilled for the classification of RA; patients with two clinical diagnoses are not excluded

Table 2.5 The 1987 ARA criteria for RA

(1) Morning stiffness	Morning stiffness in and around the joints lasting one hour before maximal movement
(2) Arthritis in three or more joint areas*	Soft tissue swelling of fluid (not bony overgrowth) observed by a physician, present simultaneously for at least six weeks
(3) Arthritis of hand joints	Swelling of wrist, MCP or PIP joints for at least six weeks
(4) Symmetrical arthritis	Simultaneous involvement of the same joint areas (defined in (2)) on both sides of the body (bilateral involvement of PIP, MCP or MTP joints is acceptable without absolute symmetry) for at least six weeks
(5) Rheumatoid nodules	Subcutaneous nodules over body prominences, extensor surfaces or in juxta-articular regions, observed by a physician
(6) Rheumatoid factor	Detected by a method positive in less than 5% of normal controls
(7) Radiographic changes	Typical of RA on posteroanterior hand and wrist radiographs; it must include erosions of unequivocal bony decalcification localized in or most marked adjacent to the involved joints (OA changes alone do not qualify)

Note: *Possible areas: right or left PIP, MCP, wrist, elbow, knee, ankle, MTP.
Key: PIP = proximal interphalangeal joints; MCP = metacarpophalangeal joints; MTP = metatarsophalangeal joints – all seen in Figure 2.9.

Q2.28: How common is RA?

An estimate of the occurrence of the disease is assessed by two measures:

(1) incidence – the rate of new cases arising over a specific time period;
(2) prevalence – the number of existing cases.

Incidence

Symmons et al. (1994) carried out a unique study of RA in the UK which showed an annual incidence rate in 1990 of 36 per 100 000 women and 14 per 100 000 men. RA is rare in men under 45 years but this becomes rapidly more common with age. In women the incidence of RA rises up to 45 and remains plateaued to 75 when it declines (Figure 2.7).

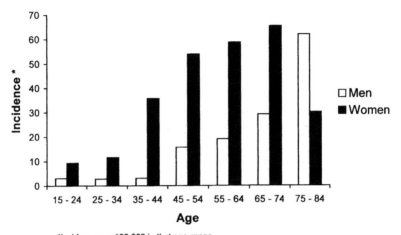

*Incidence per 100,000 in that age range

Figure 2.7 Incidence of RA.
Source: Data from Symmons et al. (1994).

Prevalence

RA is found throughout the world but it is thought to be more common in northern Europe. In the UK it can be seen in as many as 1–2% of the population (Lawrence, 1961; Spector et al., 1993). An average general practice list of 2500 patients will have between 25 and 50 patients with RA. However, this varies between practices. One rural practice in Northallerton, North Yorkshire cares for 100 RA patients, from a practice population of 6000 (Dickson, 1993), whilst Sonning Common Health Centre near Reading has 33, from a practice population of 7000 (Dargie and Proctor, 1993). In all studies, the prevalence of RA has been found to rise with age, which is to be expected in a chronic disease with a low mortality rate.

Occurrence Trends

The occurrence of RA in women appears to be in decline (Charlton et al., 1995), but the situation for men is stable. Some authors have attributed this to a protective effect of the contraceptive pill (Vandenbrouke et al., 1982). Research by Silman et al. (1983) showed that erosive, seropositive nodular RA peaked in the 1960s and subsequent generations are less severely affected. However, RA is the most common form of inflammatory joint disease in the UK with approximately one million people diagnosed.

Q2.29: Who does RA affect?

RA affects all age-groups, races and social classes and occurs in all types of climate. Although it appears in both sexes, women are affected more often than men in a ratio of about 3:1. Women aged 30–50 years are most likely to develop it, but in the very elderly RA is more common in men than women. Severity varies from a mild disease with few problems, to severe RA leading to extensive disability (Figure 2.8). About 1 in 200 women compared with 1 in 600 men have significant RA in the UK. Siblings of those with RA have a small but increased risk of developing the disease and this indicates that shared genetic or shared environmental factors contribute to the disease.

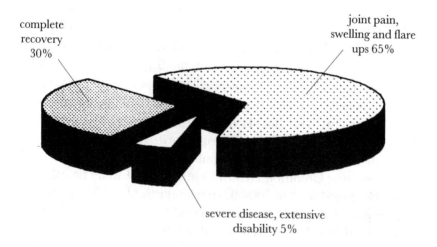

complete recovery 30%

joint pain, swelling and flare ups 65%

severe disease, extensive disability 5%

Figure 2.8 Spectrum of disease activity.

Q2.30: What causes RA?

As yet the exact causes of RA are unproven but the following factors may be implicated:

- genetic predisposition;
- reproduction and hormones;
- environment.

Genetic Factors

Although RA is not thought to be a hereditary disease, there is compelling evidence from studies of monozygotic and dizygotic twins of a strong genetic influence. This research shows a three- to fourfold increased risk of disease concordance for monozygotic twins when compared with dizygotic twins (Aho et al., 1986; Silman et al., 1993).

Genetic markers such as human leucocyte antigens (HLA) have been identified as contributing to genetic risk. Between 60% and 70% of patients with RA are HLA-DR4 positive, compared with 20% in the 'normal population'.

Reproduction and Hormonal Influences

The preponderance of women who develop RA prior to the menopause and the tendency to remission during pregnancy suggests that hormones may play an important role. Research results to date have produced conflicting results but there is evidence to suggest that the timing of the onset of RA is influenced by pregnancy. Silman et al. (1992) showed that the chances of developing RA during pregnancy are reduced, but in the first 12 months following delivery the risk increases. Breast feeding has also been implicated as an increased risk during this period (Brennen and Silman, 1994).

There is disagreement about the effects of the oral contraceptive pill on RA. One large study appeared to show that it halved the risk of developing RA, whilst others did not. A meta-analysis has shown that the contraceptive pill does not alter the risk of having RA but it may delay its onset (Spector and Hochberg, 1990).

Environment

Environmental factors include infectious agents, socioeconomic status and occupation, lifestyle and diet, although the part played by these in the development of RA remains unproven. However, anecdotal evidence suggests that environmental influences do exist (MacGregor and Silman, 1998).

Q2.31: How does RA start?

The most common form of onset is gradual and insidious, but some patients report going to bed one evening apparently fit and well and waking up the following morning unable to get out of bed. For many years it has been thought that patients whose onset is acute have a more favourable outcome than those whose onset is gradual, but the evidence for this is discordant.

Gradual onset usually starts with pain and/or stiffness in the hands, wrists or balls of the feet, which is usually symmetrical, i.e. joints on both the left and right are affected. This progresses and the joints also become swollen. A general feeling of illness ensues and patients seek help from their GP.

Q2.32: What are the signs and symptoms of RA?

RA can be preceded by a period of general ill health characterized by:

- fatigue;
- weight loss;
- anorexia.

Some patients get paraesthesia due to entrapment neuropathies. The most common site is at the wrist and is known as carpal tunnel syndrome. Pain, stiffness and synovitis involving many joints are classical, and the distribution is usually symmetrical. The most commonly affected sites and their approximate distribution are shown in Figure 2.9.

Joint effusions cause extra intra-articular pressure and when this occurs at the knee can result in Baker's cysts. If they rupture, they are sometimes misdiagnosed as venous thrombosis. RA is a disease that involves many of the bodily systems and malaise, fatigue, depression and anxiety are all commonplace.

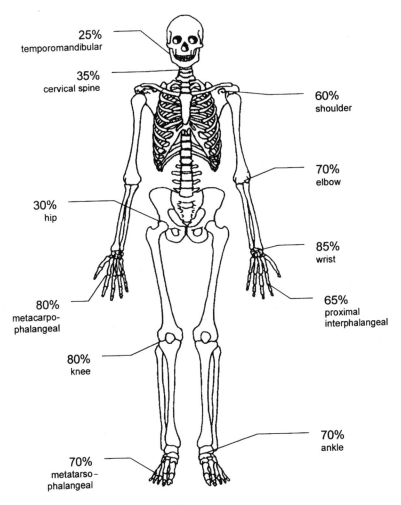

Figure 2.9 Joints commonly affected by RA.

Q2.33: What are the extra-articular features?

Other associated manifestations are common (Arthur, 1998), including:

- anaemia;
- rheumatoid nodules;
- Sjögren's syndrome;
- vasculitis;
- Felty's syndrome;

- pericarditis;
- raised liver enzymes;
- pulmonary problems;
- nerve compression.

Q2.34: What are the tests for RA?

In addition to the clinical appearance, both blood tests and X-rays aid diagnosis. They can also be used to assess disease activity.

Blood Tests

Erythrocyte sedimentation rate (ESR)

The ESR is raised when inflammation is present and is not specific to RA. It differs with sex and increases with age having a normal range of 4–20 mm/h in males and 10–25 mm/h in females. In general the ESR increases with disease activity and can reach 100 mm/h if RA is very active. It can be used in diagnosis and to monitor the efficacy of treatment.

Plasma viscosity (PV)

PV has some advantages over ESR in that it is independent of age, is not affected by red cells and it need not be processed immediately. Normal values are in the range of 1.50–1.72 cp. A level above 1.75 cp is considered to indicate active RA and if it is above 2.0 cp, severely active. It can be used in the same way as the ESR.

C-reactive protein (CRP)

The CRP is a non-specific inflammatory marker detected in the acute phase of the inflammatory response. Changes occur faster than with either the ESR or PV but levels may not rise in the presence of relatively mild inflammation. A consistently raised CRP is associated with severe RA. Normal range is 0–8 mg/l.

Rheumatoid factor (RF)

RF is an immunological investigation that proves positive in 80% of RA patients and 5% of the general population. It is an IgM/IgG immunoglobulin complex and patients with RA who have this complex are said to be sero-positive. A titre of 1:32 is classed as weakly positive and 1:64 and above indicates more active disease. Sero-positive RA is usually more aggressive than sero-negative disease producing more erosions and rheumatoid nodules.

Haemoglobin (Hb)

Patients with RA often have a low Hb and are diagnosed as having normochromic normocytic anaemia resulting from poor utilization of iron. Patients who have active RA with raised CRP, PV or ESR often have a low Hb < 10.0 g/dl attributed to their active disease. A microcytic hypochromic anaemia may indicate GI bleeding due to NSAIDs. Normal values are 13.5–18.0 g/dl in men and 11.5–16.5 g/dl in women.

Platelet count

Those with active RA often have an increased platelet count (thrombocytosis). However, lower than normal values (thrombocytopenia) can be due to side-effects of drug therapy.

X-rays

X-rays of the hands and feet are initially taken to aid diagnosis but it may take many months or even years before signs of RA are detected. The first signs usually appear in the metatarsal heads (MTPs) of the feet but in some patients erosions appear in the metacarpophalangeal joints (MCPs) of the hands. The dominant joint is usually more severely affected. Erosions look like punched-out holes on the joint margin (see Figure 2.6).

Q2.35: How is RA managed?

There is no cure for RA and so the aims of management are to:

- relieve symptoms;
- preserve/restore function;
- prevent structural damage and deformity;
- maintain a lifestyle acceptable to the patient;
- reduce psychological distress.

This is quite a task in a disease that is chronic, painful, potentially life-altering and disabling. It is an unpredictable disease that creates uncertainties for the patient, his/her partner, relatives and friends.

Many patients experience periods of exacerbation (flare) and sometimes remission occurs. When deciding on a management plan it is
important to assess the patient's physical needs but the social and
psychological implications must also be considered.

Q2.36: What treatment is available for RA?

As RA is such a multifaceted disease it may be necessary to implement many different treatment modalities. These include:

- drug therapy;
- exercise regimes;
- joint protection techniques;
- orthoses;
- complementary therapies;
- surgery;
- psychosocial support.

All of these therapies are underpinned by PE.

PE

As with OA, PE plays a central role in caring for those with RA and
there is a plethora of research to show that PE improves the patient's
physical and psychological outcome (see Chapter 4). One-to-one PE
and group PE based on the Arthritis Self Management Programme
(ASMP) are both suitable in the primary care setting.

Arthritis Care is a self-help organization that runs a number of self-
management programmes and has over 500 local branches. They and
the Arthritis Research Campaign (ARC) produce a broad range of
literature to support verbal explanation about RA and its treatments.

Drug Therapy

Drug therapy plays an important role in the treatment of RA and is
discussed in depth in Chapter 3. Three groups of medications form
the mainstay of therapy:

- analgesics;
- non-steroidal anti-inflammatory drugs (NSAIDs);
- disease-modifying anti-rheumatic drugs (DMARDs).

The first two groups relieve the symptoms of RA, but DMARDs suppress the disease itself and some patients go into remission. DMARDs are potentially toxic and require special monitoring, which is discussed in Chapter 3.

Corticosteroids can bring rapid symptom relief but they can also cause harm and so are given at low doses as sparingly as possible. Intra-articular steroids are used to good effect in both large and small joints and intramuscular (IM) Depo-Medrone is very efficacious, particularly during a 'flare'.

These categories of drugs can be used in combination without adverse drug interaction.

Physiotherapy

Exercise plays an important role in the treatment of RA. Muscle wasting and reduced range of movement can lead to functional disability and flexion deformities surprisingly quickly. A daily exercise programme (see Q5.8) will help to overcome difficulties, but this can be painful and boring for the patient. The community nurse can encourage patients in their endeavours when they attend for routine drug monitoring or during home visits. Nurses are practical people and they can suggest ways of integrating exercises into routine daily activities.

Joint Protection

The aim of joint protection is to prevent damage to vulnerable inflamed joints by reducing stresses and overuse. The occupational therapist will normally undertake an 'aids to daily living assessment' on each patient and provide splints and aids for the home (see Q5.20 and Q5.21). Patients may need to alter the way they perform certain tasks such as lifting, getting out of a chair or even preparing food, to reduce the amount of stress they place on their joints.

Footwear and Walking Aids

MTP involvement is very common in RA and patients often develop callosities in this area. The podiatrist is an invaluable member of the multidisciplinary team who can help to solve foot problems by

providing specialist footcare, footwear and orthoses (see Q5.26 and
Q5.27).

Walking aids can be helpful, but patients with multiple joint
involvement may need a walking aid with a special moulded handled
such as a Fisher stick to accommodate a painful rheumatoid hand
(see Q5.19 and Figure 5.2).

Relaxation, Dietary Advice and Complementary Therapy

As with OA all these therapies can be useful (see Q2.12, Q5.15,
Q5.28 and Q5.29).

Surgery

In RA surgery is usually undertaken:

- to relieve pain;
- to restore or improve function;
- to correct deformity;
- for cosmesis.

Most surgical interventions are elective but indications for urgent
treatment are septic arthritis, ruptured tendons and compression of
nerves and spinal cord. Common procedures are listed in Table 2.6.

Psychosocial Support

Patients with a disfiguring debilitating disease such as RA will
certainly need psychosocial support. They may be anxious and
depressed upon hearing their diagnosis and have fears for their job
or their ability to undertake household duties. The primary care
nurse can do much to help and reassure them and all these aspects
are discussed in Chapter 6.

Case Study

*Joyce is a 52-year-old happily married housewife, with an adult married daugh-
ter who lives close by. RA came on gradually soon after the birth of her daughter.
She began to feel generally tired and unwell but put this down to the increased*

Table 2.6 Common surgical procedures for RA

Procedure	Example
(1) Arthroplasty – surgical reconstruction, two types:	
(a) Excision arthroplasty. Ends of articulating surface removed leaving a gap that fills with fibrous tissue	Girdlestone arthroplasty of hip Fowlers operation – excision of MTP heads
(b) Replacement arthroplasty. Replacement of whole or part of a joint with an artificial prothesis	Total hip replacement Total knee replacement Silastic implants to replace MCPs
(2) Synovectomy – excision of excess synovial lining	Commonly undertaken on the knee and wrist
(3) Tendon repair – for ruptured tendons	Usually occurs at the fingers resulting in a 'dropped finger'
(4) Arthrodesis – surgical fixation for stability and pain relief	Fused wrist Base of thumb Atlantoaxial subluxation of the cervical spine
(5) Reconstruction of joint deformities	Swan neck deformity Ulnar drift
(6) Decompression surgery	Carpal tunnel release

workload of caring for her baby. Her joints felt stiff in the mornings and the balls of her feet and knuckles of her hands were becoming painful and swollen. After about eight months she began to lose weight and started to become stiff if she sat down to rest; her knees and wrists were swollen and painful.

Joyce decided to see her GP, who examined her joints and took blood tests for a full blood count, CRP, PV and RF, and arranged for X-rays to be taken. The CRP was raised at 40 mg/l, PV was 1.86 cp and RF 1:64. Although there were no erosions on her hands and feet she was diagnosed as having RA. Joyce was prescribed an NSAID with intermittent analgesics when necessary and referred to her local consultant rheumatologist who commenced sulphasalazine. During monitoring visits at the health centre she was taught about her disease and its treatments, and appointments were made with the physiotherapist and occupational therapist. After 12 weeks the disease activity subsided and she was monitored three-monthly at the surgery with occasional consultations at the local hospital.

Joyce was well controlled for a further five years with some changes to her NSAIDs and analgesics, but then started to have frequent flares that gradually increased in their severity and she developed nodules. She was referred back to the rheumatologist for a review of her DMARD and given Depo-Medrone 120 mg IM to settle her present symptoms. The rheumatologist commenced methotrexate (MTX) following chest X-rays and baseline liver function tests. The hospital-based clinical nurse specialist had talked to Joyce about MTX and its side-effects and also discussed these with the health centre. Joyce was then returned to the care of the health centre for monitoring. Continuity of care between the surgery and the hospital was assured by the use of a shared-care card on which blood test results and investigations were recorded, as were any changes to treatment.

The MTX appeared to help enormously, but even though she wore her sleeping splints and carried out daily exercises she developed severe erosions at the MCP joints which resulted in painful joint destruction and severe ulnar drift. Joyce eventually had silastic implants that left her hands pain free and improved her functional ability.

She became a member of her local Arthritis Care group and has helped many others come to terms with their disease and get the most out of their lives. Her latest venture has been to undertake the Patient Partners course and she now acts as a human model, teaching student doctors and health professionals about RA and its effects.

Some Common Questions

Q2.37: How will I know the difference between RA and OA?

RA is an inflammatory disease of the synovium affecting many joints and systems, making patients feel generally ill. OA affects the cartilage and normally affects only one or two joints. Although patients with OA are in pain they do not feel ill.

Q2.38: Can I tell the difference between RA and OA by looking at the blood results?

Patients with OA would not normally have any changes in their blood results, although one should be aware that NSAIDs could cause GI bleeding and thus look for a falling Hb. Those with active RA would usually have elevated levels of PV, CRP and ESR. They may also have a low Hb, raised platelet count and liver function tests (LFTs). Their RF can often be positive.

Q2.39: How will I know from the blood results which drug is helping the patient?

Analgesics, NSAIDs and DMARDs all help to lessen the symptoms of RA but only the DMARDs will alter the blood results and put the patient into remission. If the DMARD is working, elevated markers such as PV, ESR, CRP and platelets fall towards normal levels and low Hb should improve. Analgesics and NSAIDs will reduce pain and stiffness but have no effect on the actual disease and so biochemical markers will remain unchanged.

Q2.40: How will I know if the patient is in a flare?

The first sign is increasing length of morning stiffness, followed by increased pain and severe fatigue. Patients should be advised to take more rest whilst still practising a gentle exercise regime. Advise them to wear joint splints, if supplied, but to take them off every couple of hours and do a range of motion exercises.

Review their drug therapy, ensuring compliance, and to the maximum dose if necessary. Tell them to try heat or cold on any particularly bad joint and if necessary refer to the GP to arrange a Depo-Medrone injection.

Q2.41: Who should I refer to if the patient appears with a dropped tendon?

Refer them, via the GP, as soon as possible to the surgeon for tendon repair.

Q2.42: At what stage should the physiotherapist and occupational therapist be involved?

As soon as the patient has a positive diagnosis.

Q2.43: What do I say to a patient who asks about pregnancy?

There is no reason for patients not to have children. However, if they have a large family already it can be very difficult to cope. Seventy-five per cent of women who have RA improve during their pregnancy but it tends to come back with a vengeance within a few months of giving birth. There are some drugs that are contra-indicated during pregnancy and this needs full discussion (see Q3.16, Q3.39, Table 3.8, Q6.21–6.24).

Gout

Gout is one of the oldest diseases known to man and was well described by Hippocrates in the fifth century BC. It is an excruciatingly painful disease but is both treatable and preventable. The majority of cases are managed in the primary care setting but cases sometimes crop up in hospital as attacks can be precipitated by diuretics and stresses such as ketosis, acute infection or surgery (Snaith, 1996). Gout results in significant short-term disability, occupational limitations and the use of medical facilities, marking it as a significant health problem.

Q2.44: What are the pathological features of gout?

Gout is the deposition of monosodium urate crystals, chiefly in connective tissue, commonly in and around synovial joints. This occurs because of high levels of urate in the blood (hyperuricaemia), but not everyone with hyperuricaemia will develop gout. Uric acid appears in the plasma as a salt called urate and at high levels of concentration urate crystals form that shed into the joints. Repeated attacks can damage the joint and leave bony erosions associated with tophi formation; a lump of solid urate visible over joints (Figure 2.10). Occasionally calculi form in the kidneys.

Q2.45: How common is gout?

There was a 30% increase in gout between 1970 and 1982 affecting both sexes at all ages (Symmons and Bankhead, 1994). Although the incidence is rising the prevalence of chronic tophaceous gout is falling owing to improved treatment. It has been estimated that in a practice of 2000 patients 15 men and 3 women will have a tendency to gout (Snaith, 1996).

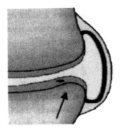
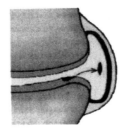
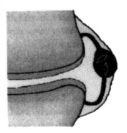

Small asymptomatic crystal deposits form in the cartilage

Crystals shed into the joint space

Free crystals cause acute inflammation of the synovium

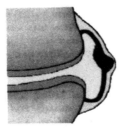
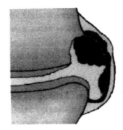

Larger deposits form

Chronic inflammatory changes occur in soft tissues and bone destruction occurs

Figure 2.10 Stages in the development of gout. Reproduced with kind permission of Geoff Hill.

Q2.46: Who does it affect?

Gout is the most common form of inflammatory arthropathy in males over age 40, the peak age of onset being between 40 and 50 years. These men usually:

- are intelligent;
- are mild/moderately obese;
- have a high intake of beer.

Women are rarely affected before the menopause and do not usually develop gout until they are over 60 years of age.

Q2.47: What are the causes of gout?

Gout is a disorder of purine metabolism leading to hyperuricaemia, which has both endogenous and exogenous causes (Table 2.7). Purine compounds are a source of nitrogen derived from cells in the foods rich in nuclei, such as yeast, liver and kidney.

Table 2.7 Causes of hyperuricaemia

Endogenous	Exogenous
Family history	Dietary purines
Obesity	Drugs
Hypertension	Alcohol
Renal function	
Hyperlipidaemia	

The higher the levels of urate the greater the risk of developing gout. The increase in the number of cases is thought to be iatrogenic (Table 2.8), the prescription of diuretics playing a major role.

Table 2.8 Drugs affecting plasma urate concentration

Salicylates
Thiazides
Frusemide
Pyrazinamide

Q2.48: How does gout present?

There are four distinct clinical phases of gout:

(1) symptomless hyperuricaemia phase;
(2) acute attack of gout;
(3) intercritical phase – phase between episodes of gout;
(4) chronic tophaceous gout.

The Acute Attack of Gout

The typical acute attack starts in the middle of the night in one big toe (first MTP joint). Within hours the toe is inflamed, swollen and excruciatingly painful; even the touch of a sheet results in unbearable pain. The attack usually reaches its peak within 24 hours, lasting for 1–3 days. During this time the patient may have a slight fever with malaise and the skin of the toe may peel. If untreated the attack will settle and the joint will return to normal within two weeks.

About 50% of first attacks and 70% of all attacks occur in the first MTP joint and 90% are monarticular. However, gout does affect other sites including the:

- ankle   (15%);
- mid-tarsal   (15%);
- fingers   (15%);
- knee   (10%);
- wrist   (5%);
- elbow   (5%).

Chronic Tophaceous Gout

Thanks to the advent of effective hyperuricaemia therapy this condition is now relatively rare. Chronic gout results in gross destructive joint disease accompanied by subcutaneous tophi and olecranon bursitis. Tophi do not usually develop until gout has been present for about 10 years and although they can appear at any site they are most common on the fingers, toes and the lobes of the ear. Tophi cause local inflammation and can ulcerate and exude a white chalky material. They can also become infected.

Q2.49: What are the tests for gout?

Tests include laboratory investigations and X-rays.

1 Blood tests. Baseline investigations include urea, creatinine and fasting lipids, which may be abnormal. Because of the inflammatory component there is likely to be some leucocytosis and varying degrees of elevation of the ESR, PV and CRP. LFT results may be elevated owing to alcohol consumption, particularly æ-glutamyl transferase.

2 Urate level. The urate level is almost always elevated during an acute attack and in chronic gout. Normal values are 210–420μmol/1(3.5–7mg/100 ml) adult males and 170–360μmol/1

(2.8–6 mg/100 ml) in females. The risk of gout increases considerably with concentrations over 600μmol/1 (10 mg/100 ml). In chronic tophaceous gout the levels can be 50 or 100 times normal.

3 Synovial fluid. If possible a sample of synovial fluid should be examined under polarized light. In acute gout the fluid is thin and murky and contains polymorphonuclear cells and, most significantly, urate crystals. Although the inflammation is less marked in tophaceous gout, crystals are still found in the joint or bursal fluid.

4 X-rays. Acute gout shows soft tissue swelling but in chronic gout X-ray shows:

- narrowing of the joint space;
- sclerosis;
- bone cysts;
- erosions.

Q2.50 How is gout managed?

The principal goals of treatment are to treat acute attacks early and effectively, and to correct the causative hyperuricaemia. Acute gout is treated by:

- inhibiting inflammation, through drug therapy;
- rest.

The earlier drug therapy is started, the quicker the attack will resolve (see Q3.43). Although extremely painful, acute gout is a self-limiting condition and treatment for reduction of uric acid levels is contraindicated until the attack has resolved.

Rest

Rest will aid recovery and as the majority of patients are unable to weight bear, bed rest is the most practical option. The joint can be protected from the weight of bedcovers by use of a cage.

Q2.51: How can gout be prevented?

Gout can be prevented by correcting hyperuricaemia by restoring urate levels to < 360μmol/1 (6 mg/100 ml). Lower levels are necessary to achieve resorption of tophi. This can be achieved by:

- adjusting contributing factors;
- drug therapy.

Adjusting Contributing Factors

A number of factors that contribute to hyperuricaemia are correctable (Table 2.9). A low purine diet can reduce previous levels by 15% (see Q5.33) but this is difficult to sustain for long periods. An increase in urinary excretion reduces it by rather more (Figure 2.11) and simply losing a few pounds can facilitate this. Other adjustments include:

- reduction of alcohol consumption;
- removal of diuretics wherever possible;
- treatment of hypertension.

Table 2.9 Factors contributing to hyperuricaemia

Obesity
Regular consumption of alcohol
Diuretic therapy
Hypertension
High consumption of dietary purines
Hypertriglyceridemia
Low urinary flow

Drug therapy

Drugs used in the treatment of hyperuricaemia have to be taken for life. There is widespread agreement on the indications for the commencement of therapy (Table 2.10).

Two types of drugs are used:

(1) uricosuric drugs: increase urate excretion;
(2) xanthine oxidase inhibitors: reduce urate production;
(see Q3.44).

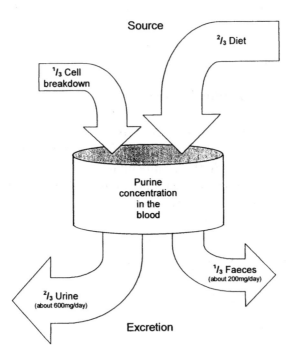

Figure 2.11 Purine metabolism.

Table 2.10 Indications for commencing hypouricaemic drugs

Three or more acute attacks of gout
Tophi
Bone/cartilage destruction
Gout and kidney disease
Urolithiasis (kidney stones)
High urate levels

Q2.52: Is PE important?

Teaching about the disease and its treatments plays a vital role in patient care as changes in lifestyle and lifelong therapy may be necessary. Patients need to be aware of the early signs and symptoms of an approaching attack so that they can begin treatment immediately.

Case Study

*Michael is a 55-year-old man who has a small catering company. He is over-
weight and has a history of hypertension. He has been feeling tired with some
vague aches and pains which he has put down to the extra workload of the
Christmas period. He was awakened at 2 a.m. by pain in his left great toe
that was increasing by the hour. As the pain became very severe he started to
feel as though he had a fever, began shivering and then felt chilled. He spent a
terrible night and was unable to sleep because of the pain; even the weight of a
sheet on his toe was unbearable. By the morning the toe looked red and swollen
and his wife called his GP who suspected an acute attack of gout.*

*He was immediately started on indomethacin. Blood tests showed elevated
urate levels of 660μmol/1 (11 mg/100 ml) and CRP, but no other problems.
The indomethacin helped to resolve the pain to bearable levels in two days, but
the episode took about 10 days to resolve fully.*

*Michael attended the surgery for a follow-up appointment at which his
blood pressure was checked and found to be elevated. His drug therapy was
increased, which controlled his hypertension. He was given dietary advice and
managed to reduce his weight by 20 lb over the ensuing months by restricting
his calorie intake and alcohol consumption. He has had one further attack, but
was able to limit its severity by immediately starting indomethacin.*

Some Common Questions

Q2.53: Does heavy drinking cause gout?

No, but it can bring on an acute attack.

Q2.54: Do acute attacks of gout cause joint destruction?

The joint returns to its normal state after an acute attack. It is only if
the disease is left untreated after a number of attacks that erosions
and deformity are caused.

Q2.55: What analgesics can patients with gout take?

Almost everyone needs an analgesic occasionally, be it for a
headache or mild aches and pains. Paracetamol is fine but any drug
containing aspirin should be avoided even in small doses, as this
affects urate excretion and can precipitate an attack.

Q2.56: Are there any drugs that interact with allopurinol?

Co-administration of ampicillin produces a threefold increase of the risk of developing a skin rash.

Q2.57: Is gout associated with any other diseases?

Patients with gout often have undiagnosed hypertension and/or cardiac disease and thus, when the patient visits the surgery after his/her first attack, he/she should be fully investigated.

Q2.58: What is the most common side-effect of hypouricaemic therapy?

Gastric upsets and rashes, but in general such therapy is remarkably safe and well tolerated.

Q2.59: Why do NSAIDs help acute gout?

They are not a cure for gout, but they do help to reduce the symptoms by reducing the inflammation and swelling, which lessens the pain.

Q 2.60: Can anything else help?

Drinking lots of fluid during an attack and between attacks will help to get rid of urate through the kidneys.

Osteoporosis

In 1994 the World Health Organization defined osteoporosis as a disease characterized by low bone mass and microarchitectural deterioration of bone tissue, leading to enhanced bone fragility and a consequent increase in fracture risk (Figure 2.12).

Osteoporosis has become an increasingly important public health problem and it is responsible for significant morbidity and mortality. The cost in human terms is not quantifiable and the financial cost in the country is £740 million per annum (Compston and Rosen, 1997).

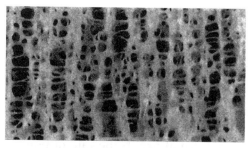

Normal bone

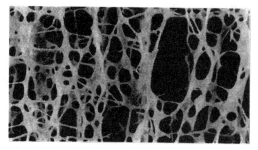

Osteoporotic bone

Figure 2.12 Osteoporotic bone compared with normal bone. Reproduced with kind permission of Professor Alan Boyd.

Q2.61: What are the pathological features of osteoporosis?

Cortical and trabecular bone becomes osteopenic and susceptible to fracture as a result of loss of bone mineral and hydroxyapatite. Bone turnover is reduced and there is a negative calcium balance.

Q2.62: How common is osteoporosis?

This depends on whether osteoporosis is defined on the basis of bone mass alone or whether fracture is a prerequisite for the disorder (Cooper, 1993). Osteoporosis affects one in four women (one in two over the age of 70), and one in 12 men.

Q2.63: What are the most commonly affected sites?

In the UK the most commonly affected sites are recorded as an annual incidence of fractures: 60 000 hip, 50 000 wrist, 40 000 vertebral (Compston and Rosen, 1997).

Q2.64: What is normal bone health and peak bone mass?

Bone is a living tissue that continually remodels throughout life. This enables the skeleton to grow in childhood, respond to physical stresses and repair structural damage resulting from trauma. The adult skeleton comprises 80% cortical and 20% trabecular bone. Cortical bone is predominantly found in the shafts of long bones whilst trabecular bone is situated in the vertebrae, pelvis and the end of long bones. In normal health the rate of bone formation equals the rate of bone reabsorption, a process known as coupling. The three major cells involved in this process are:

- osteoclasts: to reabsorb bone;
- osteoblasts: to synthesize and build bone matrix;
- osteocytes: involved in the communication process
                     influencing bone modelling.

Bone modelling is initiated by a period of reabsorption lasting about two weeks. The osteoclasts erode an area of bone, attracting osteoblasts to the reabsorption cavity. New bone is deposited in this area over the next three months (see Figure 2.13).

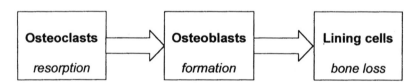

Figure 2.13 Bone turnover.

Throughout life bone is constantly being absorbed and replaced. It continues to grow until about 20 and peak bone mass is usually achieved around age 25–35 years. Involuntary bone loss starts between the age of 35 and 40. Women lose 35–50% of trabecular bone and 25–30% of cortical bone over their lifetime, and men lose 15–45% of trabecular bone and 5–10% of cortical bone over their life span. Peak bone mass is the same in both sexes but following the menopause, women lose bone mass much faster than men.

In the United States 45% of women aged 50 or older have low bone mass at one of the three major sites:

- lumbar spine;
- proximal femur;
- radius.

These data suggest that as many as 2.4 million British women have a bone mass lower than one would expect for the age of the patient (Cooper, 1993).

Q 2.65: What are the features of osteoporotic fractures?

Osteoporotic fractures show four distinct features:

(1) incidence rates are greater in women than men;
(2) rates increase with age;
(3) they occur at trabecular bone sites;
(4) they occur with minimal trauma.

Common sites at which fractures occur are shown in Figure 2.14.

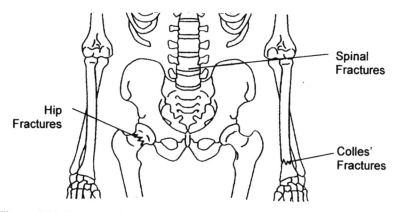

Figure 2.14 Common sites of osteoporotic fractures.

Hip Fractures

The most severe osteoporotic fractures occur at the hip, usually following an indoor fall, although they can occur spontaneously. Some 90% of hip fractures happen over the age of 50 and 80% are in women (Gallagher et al., 1980). About one-third of people become totally dependent on others for activities of daily living following a hip fracture. The mortality rate is 10–20% (Melton, 1988) and the majority of deaths occur within six months of the fracture, with a higher incidence in men with co-morbidity.

Vertebral Fractures

In women, rates of vertebral fracture are higher than hip fractures under age 70 but not after this age. The overall age adjusted incidence in women is 1.9 times greater than in men (Cooper et al., 1992).

Radial Fractures

These fractures usually occur after a fall on the outstretched arm. In women incidence rates increase linearly between 40 and 65 years and then stabilize. In men the incidence rate remains constant between 20 and 80 years.

Q2.66: What factors influence bone mass?

There are six factors that affect bone mass:

(1) genetics;
(2) exercise;
(3) diet;
(4) smoking and alcohol;
(5) low body weight;
(6) hormones.

1 Genetic factors. Genetic influences account for as much as 80% of the variance in peak bone mass (Slemenda et al., 1991). Negroid populations have a higher bone mass than Caucasians or Asians and men have bigger skeletons than women, with a higher bone density due to bone size. Daughters of mothers with osteoporosis have lower than expected peak bone density.

2 Exercise. Physical activity and strength may explain up to 40% of the variance in adult bone density (Pocock et al., 1986). Bone mass is greater in young children and adults who exercise regularly than in their less active counterparts (Nilsson and Westlin, 1971).

(3) Diet. Long-term calcium intake in both men and women has an influence on the attainment or maintenance of peak bone mass. Table 2.11 shows the recommended daily intake of calcium for different age-groups.

Table 2.11 Commonly recommended daily intake of calcium

Age/sex	Daily intake (mg)
Children 7–10 years	550
Males 11–18 years	1000
Females 11–18 years	800
Adult male	700–1000
Adult female	700–1000
Pregnant females	700

(4) Smoking and alcohol consumption. Smoking can lead to an early menopause and also reduce body weight. Excessive alcohol consumption can have an adverse effect on the skeleton, though it is uncertain whether this is due to an effect on peak bone mass or the subsequent rate of bone loss.

5 Low body weight. The loss of bone is more rapid in women with low body weight. The protective effects of high body weight on the skeleton may be due to the mechanical effects of body weight on bone formation and the increased production of oestrone in fat (Christiansen et al., 1987).

6 Hormonal factors. An early menarche, pregnancy and, in some cases, the use of oral contraceptive pill are all associated with increased bone mass (Goldsmith and Johnston, 1975). The cessation of oestrogen production following the menopause has the biggest influence on reducing bone mass.

Q2.67: What causes osteoporosis?

Osteoporosis is classified as being primary or secondary. Primary causes include:

- ageing;
- menopause;
- low adult bone density.

One in 10 women and four in 10 men are at risk of developing osteoporosis as a result of other conditions (see Table 2.12).

Table 2.12 Risk factors in the development of osteoporosis

Premature (under the age of 45), natural, surgical or radiation-induced menopause
Long-term use of steroid treatment
Cushing's syndrome
Secondary oestrogen deficiency, e.g. anorexia nervosa
Previous low-trauma fracture
Family history
Gastrectomy
Immobilizing diseases
Excessive alcohol consumption

Q2.68: How is osteoporosis identified?

In many people osteoporosis remains the silent epidemic and a person may not be aware that he/she has the condition until he/she experiences a fracture. However, the condition can be identified by:

- dual energy X-ray absorptiometry (DEXA);
- quantitative computed tomography (QCT);
- ultrasound measurements;
- radiology.

DEXA

DEXA is a safe, non-invasive technique that is currently the most precise and widely used method of assessing bone density and the best predictor of fracture rate. The Department of Health recommends that individuals at high risk of osteoporosis should have access to bone densitometry (Barlow, 1994). Those at risk include individuals with:

- oestrogen deficiency – particularly after natural or surgical menopause, or prolonged amenorrhoea;
- vertebral deformity – multiple low-trauma fractures or osteopenia as noted on X-rays;
- certain treatments – such as bisphosphonates, where response is less predictable and the effect of such intervention can be monitored;
- long-term corticosteroid use – including individuals who have received or are likely to receive a dose of over 5 mg daily for more than three months. Decisions about the introduction of

steroid-sparing or bone-protecting agents can be facilitated following the DEXA.

QCT

This estimates bone mineral content, allowing cortical bone to be distinguished from trabecular bone. However, it is expensive and it exposes patients to radiation.

Ultrasound measurements

Ultrasound measurements of the calcaneum are currently being evaluated as a means of measuring bone density.

Radiology

X-rays are the best method of documenting fractures but are of no use in the early detection of osteoporosis as 30% of the skeletal density may be lost before it is apparent on X-ray.

Q 2.69: What are the signs and symptoms of osteoporosis?

Symptoms of osteoporosis do not usually present until patients sustain a fracture and then the immediate effect is severe pain. Symptomatology includes:

- severe pain;
- fracture;
- thoracic kyphosis (Figure 2.15) due to vertebral fractures, resulting in height loss;
- breathlessness.

Q2.70: What is the recommended management of osteoporosis?

The goals of management are to:

- prevent fractures;
- reduce pain;
- minimize disability;
- improve the quality of life.

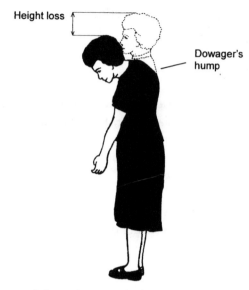

Figure 2.15 Dowager's hump in osteoporosis.

Preventive drug therapy is the introduction of either hormone replacement therapy (HRT) or antiresorptive agents.

HRT: It has been shown that HRT prevents bone loss and fracture in post-menopausal women.

Antiresorptive agents: These agents decrease bone reabsorption and include:

- bisphosphonates;
- calcium supplements;
- calcitonin;
- vitamin D;
- vitamin D metabolites;
- anabolic agents.

For explanation of the above see Q3.45.

Other treatments include:

- analgesia (see Chapter 3);
- physiotherapy (see Chapter 5);
- hydrotherapy (see Q5.17);

- dietary advice (see Q5.32);
- PE (see Q4.2).

Community nurses can do much to both prevent and minimize the effects of osteoporosis. For instance, Voyce (1998) suggests that:

- Midwives can advise pregnant, lactating and weaning mothers on the importance of good nutrition, plenty of calcium and a healthy lifestyle.
- Health visitors should stress the importance of adequate calcium in the diet and the importance of exercise for children aged one upwards.
- School nurses, practice nurses and health visitors can advise schoolchildren directly about the effects of diet and exercise and their relationship to peak bone mass.
- The key role of district nurses in promoting the health of housebound men and women must not be ignored.

Some Common Questions

Q2.71: Can anything be done to prevent osteoporosis?

Yes, there are a number of preventive measures including:

- regular exercise;
- an adequate intake of calcium and vitamin D (see Q5.32);
- a safe home environment to minimize the likelihood of falls;
- not smoking;
- not drinking alcohol to excess.

Q2.72: What can I do to prevent patients from falling and fracturing themselves?

Consideration of predisposing factors such as drowsiness due to drugs, postural hypotension and poor eyesight can help to eliminate falls. For example, patients at risk could be referred to a physiotherapist to improve their balance, while simple aids such as a walking stick can reduce the chance of falling. The home environment can be assessed for loose rugs and cables, which cause many unnecessary falls.

Q2.73: Are there any aids to reduce the impact of falls?

Yes, specially designed hip protectors that absorb the impact on falling have been shown to reduce the incidence of hip fractures. These are usually available via an occupational therapist.

Q2.74: Are there any patients who should not take HRT?

Women should not be prescribed HRT if they have had:

• cancer of the breast or uterus;
• recent blood clots;
• liver damage;
• kidney disease – requires specialist advice.

Q2.75: Why is there a low uptake of HRT in the UK?

Several reasons influence whether women will commence HRT including:

• a desire to avoid unnecessary drugs;
• a wish not to have to take hormones;
• fear of side-effects;
• anxiety about breast cancer;
• the dislike of continuing with periods which occurs with some preparations.

Many of these fears can be overcome with counselling or PE.

Q2.76: Where can I obtain more information?

The National Osteoporosis Society (NOS) produces evidence-based educational material for both health professionals and patients. Their address is given in Chapter 7.

Fibromyalgia

Fibromyalgia is a common condition characterized by both physical and psychological distress. It is typically associated with:

• widespread skeletal pain;

- persistent fatigue;
- non-refreshing sleep;
- generalized stiffness.

The prognosis for fibromyalgia is often poor. One study found that five years after diagnosis 50% of patients reported an increase in their original symptoms (Henriksson, 1994). Although the aetiology remains unknown the objective is clearly to minimize the impact of the symptoms on everyday life. Nurses can begin the process of enabling patients to develop effective coping skills by offering advice on pain control, exercise, sleep and other aspects of lifestyle adaptation.

Q2.77: Who does fibromyalgia affect?

The condition occurs primarily in women aged between 25 and 45 years and affects 3.4% of women and 0.5% of men (Wolfe et al., 1995); the female preponderance is approximately 90%.

Q2.78: What causes fibromyalgia?

The aetiology and pathogenesis of fibromyalgia are unknown but are likely to include more than one factor. Greenfield et al. (1992) refer to the possibility of triggers, such as a whiplash injury or infection, that activate a pre-existing abnormality. Investigations have been carried out into alterations in:

- neurotransmitter regulations;
- immune system function;
- sleep physiology;
- hormonal control mechanisms.

Q2.79: How does fibromyalgia affect sleep?

Patients with fibromyalgia typically experience a cycle of sleep disturbance and pain (Figure 2.16). In some patients the condition has been associated with an electroencephalogram abnormality called alpha-delta sleep which may interfere with circadian secretions of pituitary hormone and lead to feelings of unrefreshed sleep. One study has highlighted the possibility of a disruption of the growth hormone somatomedin C (Bennet et al., 1992) and other

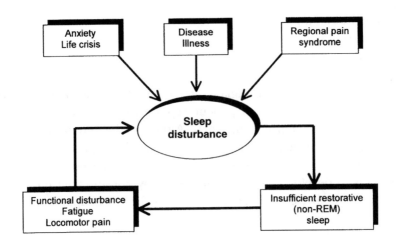

Figure 2.16 Sleep disturbance in fibromyalgia.

abnormalities of the neuroendocrine axis to explain both the sleep
disorder and the pain of fibromyalgia.

Q2.80: Are muscle studies useful?

Muscle biopsies, serum levels of muscle enzymes, electromyography,
exercise testing and nuclear magnetic resonance have failed to show
any global defect of muscle metabolism in fibromyalgia patients
(Durelte et al., 1991).

Q2.81: How do psychological factors affect fibromyalgia?

Patients with fibromyalgia often exhibit signs of depression. It is difficult to conclude whether the depression causes fibromyalgia or
whether depression is a feature of the condition.

Q2.82: How is fibromyalgia diagnosed?

The American College of Rheumatology criteria for the classification of fibromyalgia (Wolfe, 1990) include:

(1) a history of widespread pain, usually in all four quadrants of the
    body. Skeletal pain can also be present and may include areas such
    as the cervical spine, anterior chest, thoracic spine and lower back;

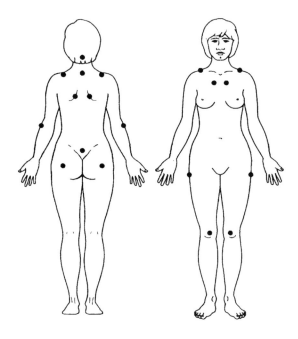

Figure 2.17 Tender points used to assess fibromyalgia.

(2) the presence of multiple hyperanalgesic tender points (Figure 2.17). A tender point is determined by digital palpation using firm pressure. A tender point has to be painful at palpation and not just tender. For a diagnosis of fibromyalgia, pain has to be experienced in 11 of the tender points.

Q2.83: What are the associated symptoms?

Fibromyalgia is associated with many symptoms, both physical and psychological (Table 2.13) and it can also accompany other conditions. Patients with SLE often experience fibromyalgia-type symptoms that present them with problems coping with their condition. Symptoms of myalgic encephalomyelitis (ME) overlap many of those of fibromyalgia. However, the dominant symptom is fatigue and patients can often recall a viral infection prior to the advent of their condition.

Table 2.13 Symptoms associated with fibromyalgia

Physical manifestations:

Irritable bladder
Irritable bowel
Migraines
Muscle spasms
Dizziness
Feelings of swelling
Lack of endurance
Numbness and tingling
Sore throat
Stiffness
Swollen glands
Tension headaches
Temperature changes
Raynaud's phenomena
Dysmenorrhoea

Psychological manifestations:

Anxiety
Confusion
Mood swings
Irritability
Memory blanks
Panic attacks
Word mix-ups
Trouble concentrating

Q2.84: How is fibromyalgia managed?

Patients with this condition often remain in primary care and only access secondary care for confirmation of their diagnosis from the rheumatologist. The main aim is to enable the patient and his/her family to adopt positive coping strategies (Ryan, 1995b). Unfortunately there is no quick fix and the patient will require the nurse to provide:

- support;
- education;
- guidance.

Interventions should include:

- PE – teaching about the syndrome;
- pain control;
- exercise;
- advice about concentration and memory recall;
- stress reduction.

PE

Taking the time to teach about the syndrome and its effects may be very beneficial to these patients. They may have had the condition for a number of years and been given no diagnosis; just being 'believed' can be an enormous relief and help. Both PE and exercise are helpful but a combination of the two has been shown to be more beneficial than either one or no intervention (Burckhardt et al., 1994).

Pain Control

Drugs such as analgesics have a limited role in this condition and thus pain management programmes are best focused on changing the patient's perceptions about his/her pain. The utilization of behavioural interventions such as relaxation and yoga will enable patients to regain control over their condition.

Sleep

Somehow the feeling of exhaustion must be overcome and to aid restorative sleep is a prime objective of management. It is important that the patient develops a nightly routine and adheres strictly to it. The environment should be prepared with a comfortable mattress, appropriate pillows and distracting noises blocked out. A warm bath before settling can enhance relaxation. Stimulants such as tea, coffee or alcohol should not be taken late at night and nasal decongestants should be avoided. Some patients will benefit from a nightly low dose of amitriptyline as this modifies pain and aids sleep (see Q3.5). This medication needs to be taken for three months before its effectiveness can be assessed.

Exercise

Exercise needs to be planned and carried out each day and patients need to be informed that initially it can increase pain and fatigue as inactive muscles start to function again. It is also imperative that realistic, manageable goals are agreed to prevent demotivation. Walking, swimming and aerobic exercise are excellent, and whichever are chosen should be introduced gradually.

Concentration and Memory

Distractions should be removed as these can limit the ability to concentrate and demanding mental work should be carried out at the time of the day when the individual feels most alert. Advising patients to write lists or keep a calendar can aid the memory as long as these are kept in a place where they will be viewed.

Minimizing Stress

Patients with fibromyalgia report heightened stress scores (Dailey et al., 1990), so the reduction or avoidance of stressful situations is helpful. Setting goals to identify the stressors in the patient's life can be of help, and in some cases the aid of a professional counsellor may be needed.

Some Common Questions

Q2.85: Are there any blood tests for fibromyalgia?

There are no tests specific to fibromyalgia. However, a full blood count, thyroid function tests and inflammatory markers are frequently used to exclude other reasons for the presenting symptoms. A full clinical history and musculoskeletal examination will also ensure that the symptoms are not related to another source.

Q2.86: Will diet help?

Although there is no special diet for these patients, healthy eating and weight reduction for those who are obese will aid vitality and body image.

Q2.87: Do NSAIDs help?

NSAIDs are not really helpful for the type of pain associated with fibromyalgia and it is better to stick to simple analgesics as they have fewer side-effects.

Q2.88: What other forms of pain relief are advocated?

Heat or ice packs can be helpful and some practitioners inject the tender points with local anaesthetic. Unfortunately this is not over-useful as patients with fibromyalgia have multiple tender points. TENS units are sometimes effective, as is massage.

Q2.89: Are splints useful?

A soft cervical collar for sleeping in may help to reduce neck pain.

Summary

The majority of rheumatic diseases are chronic, painful, disfiguring, disabling and incurable. Consequently they change the lives of the patients, their families and friends. Few are ever hospitalized because of their arthritis, and the majority live their lives in the community, managed by members of the primary health care team. Enabling the patient who has one of these complex diseases to achieve the maximum quality of life requires nurses to gain an in-depth knowledge of the disease, its effects and its treatments. Community nurses play a pivotal role in the care of people with these conditions, as they often stay for a number of years with a practice, where staff are accessible and approachable. This provides the time and place to build a rapport with both patient and carer, which enables the nurse to support, educate and empower them.

Chapter 3
Drug Therapy and Drug Monitoring

Drug Therapy

The role of drug therapy in patients with a rheumatological condition must be understood by nurses caring for these patients, to ensure that appropriate support can be offered.

Drug therapy has many functions. One of its main roles is to reduce pain, which is a major contributor to the morbidity, disability and social economic cost of musculoskeletal disorders (Cohen, 1994). Pain is a cardinal feature of inflammatory arthritis and is cited by both patients and rheumatologists as one of the major symptoms that interfere with daily functioning. Patients with inflammatory arthritis will often require a combination of drug treatments, not only to help with the symptoms of pain and stiffness but also to suppress the disease activity that is occurring. This will often necessitate the use of disease-modifying anti-rheumatic agents, such as gold. The administration of these medicines will be discussed in depth later in this chapter.

Patients may experience pain from the inflammation of the soft tissue or joint, or from damage to the joint and its associated structures. Acute pain, for example resulting from a sports injury, can be a transient experience, whereas chronic pain associated with fibromyalgia or rheumatoid arthritis (RA) is an ongoing experience often accompanied by symptoms of anxiety and depression. It is important to remember that whatever the nature or cause of the pain, it remains a unique, subjective personal experience for the individual concerned.

Pain receptors are situated in the tissues of the body, especially the skin, synovium of the joints and walls of the arteries. These receptors are referred to as nociceptors as they respond to noxious stimuli. Such receptors can be categorized by their stimulus:

(1) mechanical changes: in inflammatory conditions such as RA, an increase in the volume of synovial fluid in the joint cavity can cause pain by distending the capsule;
(2) temperature changes: extreme changes in temperature can stimulate receptors;
(3) inflammatory changes: the inflammatory response and the release of prostaglandin, bradykinin, histamine and serotonin will activate nociceptors.

This chapter is divided into one section for each drug classification and a section for investigations.

Section 1: Analgesia

Q3.1: What pharmacological approaches can be used in pain?

Pharmacological approaches include:

(1) non-opioid drugs;
(2) compound analgesia;
(3) opioid drugs;
(4) tricyclic drugs;
(5) non-steroidal anti-anflammatory drugs (NSAIDs).

Q3.2: When are non-opioids used?

They are used to treat patients with mild to moderate pain, and represent the first rung on the analgesia ladder. They include the medications paracetamol and aspirin, which work by blocking the synthesis and secretions of prostaglandins, preventing nociceptor sensitization.

Q3.3: What is compound analgesia?

Compound analgesia contains a fixed ratio combination of non-opioid (paracetamol) and opioid analgesia (dextropropoxyphene or codeine preparations). Compound analgesia is used to bridge the void between non-opioid and opioid analgesia. Examples include:

- Co-codamol (paracetamol and codeine);
- Co-dydramol (paracetamol and dihydrocodeine);
- Co-codaprin (codeine phosphate and aspirin);
- Co-proxamol (paracetamol and dextropropoxyphene).

Side-effects from these medications include dizziness, sedation, nausea and vomiting, constipation (especially as many patients are less functionally active) and abnormal liver function tests (LFTs).

Q3.4: When is opioid analgesia used?

Opioid analgesia is used to treat severe pain. Its role in the management of musculoskeletal conditions remains controversial (Cohen, 1994). Certain patients seem to benefit without experiencing adverse effects and addiction but the question of true efficacy has not yet been assessed (Jamison, 1996). Opioid analgesia works by slotting into the opioid receptors of the brain and spinal cord. Examples of opioid drugs and their potential side-effects are given in Tables 3.1 and 3.2.

Table 3.1 Opioid drugs

Low efficacy	High efficacy
Codeine	Buprenorphine
Dihydrocodeine	Dextromaramide
Dextropropoxyphene	Diamorphine
Nalbuphine	Dipipanone
Pentazocine	Meptazinal
	Methadone
	Morphine
	Papaveretum
	Pethidine
	Tramadol

Table 3.2 Potential side-effects of opioids

Nausea and vomiting	Bradycardia/tachycardia
Constipation	Hallucinations
Respiratory depression	Mood changes
Hypotension	Addiction
Dry mouth	Reduced libido
Micturition difficulties	

Q3.5: What are tricyclic drugs?

Tricyclic drugs, for example amitriptyline, appear to have a synergistic effect with centrally acting analgesia and the stimulation of endorphine production. They are often used in conditions such as fibromyalgia, where patients experience chronic pain, unrefreshed sleep and low mood. Side-effects with these drugs may occur initially but often settle after a month. Reactions can include sedation, dry mouth, arrthythmias and constipation.

Q3.6: What education do patients need regarding analgesia?

Patients should be advised to:

- take analgesia regularly if they are experiencing constant pain;
- take analgesia when they experience pain and before the pain increases in its intensity;
- regard over-the-counter medications with care and always consult the pharmacist before purchasing additional treatments;
- take their analgesia as prescribed to assess its efficacy;
- beware of the potential side-effects, e.g. constipation, and make dietary adjustments if possible;
- not feel guilty about taking analgesia. It is important to minimize pain to increase physical and psychological functioning.

Section 2: Non-steroidal Anti-inflammatory Drugs (NSAIDs)

Q3.7: What are NSAIDs?

NSAIDs are among the most commonly prescribed drugs in the world. Their primary objective is to reduce the cardinal symptoms of the inflammation, which include pain, stiffness, swelling and warmth. The presence of these symptoms affects all aspects of well-being. Apart from reducing inflammation, NSAIDs also possess analgesic and anti-pyretic properties to treat the associated features of inflammation. NSAIDs are classified on the basis of their chemical structure (see Table 3.3). These medications work within days of commencement and will only continue to be effective as long as the blood levels of the drug are maintained. Patients who omit their medications for any reason will often experience a recurrence of symptoms.

Table 3.3 Classification of the chemical structure of NSAIDs

Carboxylic acids	Acetylated, e.g. aspirin, non-acetylated, e.g. choline salicylate, diflunisal
Acetic acids	Indomethacin, diclofenac, sulindac, etodaloc
Propionic acids	Ibuprofen, flurbioprofen, fenbrufen, fenoprofen, ketoprofen, tiaprofenic acid
Fenamic acids	Piroxicam, phenylbutazone, azapropazone, oxyphenylbutazone, tenoxicam
Non-acidic compounds	e.g. nabumetone

Q3.8: How do you decide which NSAID to prescribe?

Research has shown a marked individual response to NSAIDs when used in patients with RA (Huskisson et al., 1974). If a patient experiences a poor response to one NSAID another one should be tried. There can be variation in response even when the NSAID is from the same chemical family, although the reason for this is not known. The ultimate goal is to choose a preparation that combines the greatest level of effectiveness with the least toxicity for each patient.

Q3.9: When are NSAIDs usually prescribed?

Patients with inflammatory conditions such as RA, ankylosing spondylitis and psoriatic arthritis may have to take these medications on a regular basis to achieve symptomatic relief.

Patients with sports injuries, pseudo gout and gout may require short-term use of an NSAID.

Q3.10: Will an NSAID help relieve pain in osteoarthritis (OA)?

Patients with OA are often better managed on simple analgesia, especially as the risks of side-effects from NSAIDs increases with age and may outweigh the anticipated potential therapeutic effect.

Q3.11: How do NSAIDs work?

NSAIDs act on many of the pathways that are involved in the production of the inflammatory response suppressing prostaglandin synthesis. When prostaglandins are induced, inflammation occurs accompanied by the associated features of warmth, erythema and oedema. Prostaglandins also have a housekeeping role, lining the stomach and influencing kidney function. When their production is suppressed by the use of an NSAID these organs are at risk. There has been great interest in the development of drugs that would inhibit the inflammatory action of prostaglandins whilst leaving their other functions intact. A new type of NSAID e.g. meloxicam has been developed, whose action is to reduce inflammation but preserve the housekeeping role of prostaglandin. It is too early to state how successful this drug will be in achieving this objective.

Q 3.12: How are NSAIDs administered?

NSAIDs can be administered orally, often in slow-release compounds to help with early-morning stiffness, which is a characteristic feature of RA, topically, intramuscularly (IM) or in suppository form.

Topical Preparations

There are only a few NSAIDs available that can be administered onto the skin. They have been shown to be more effective than placebo (Thompson and Dunne, 1995), although local skin sensitivity may occur. There is some absorption into the circulation and therefore patients should be advised to keep to the stated dose.

IM

Only a few drugs are administerd by IM injection. Ketoprofen, diclofenac and piroxicam can be given IM deep into the gluteal muscle.

Suppositories

These are often prescribed to reduce the risk of gastric irritation by the direct effect of the NSAID on the gastric mucosa. However, there is still a risk of gastric ulceration mediated via the circulation, and a possibility of rectal bleeding. For patients with reduced manual dexterity, difficulty can be experienced in removing the packaging and in the administration of the suppository.

Contraindications for taking NSAIDs are listed in Table 3.4.

Table 3.4 Contraindications for taking NSAIDs

Renal insufficiency
Hypertension
Peptic ulceration
Gastropathy

Q3.13: What advice should patients be given before commencing an NSAID?

Patients should be advised to:

- always take their NSAIDs with food;
- never take more than the stated dose (even if the pain and stiffness is heightened) without discussing this first with the doctor/nurse;
- report any symptoms of indigestion or upper gastric discomfort to the doctor/nurse;
- take care when purchasing over-the-counter medications and discuss this with the pharmacist;
- consult their doctor/nurse if the medication is not helping to reduce symptoms.

Q3.14: What are the side-effects of NSAIDs?

NSAIDs account for 25% of reported adverse reactions, 75% of which are experienced by people over 65 years of age. In general NSAIDs share a common spectrum of side-effects, although the frequency of particular side-effects varies between different compounds. Between 10% and 15% of patients will experience mild side-effects, primarily on the gastrointestinal (GI) system. Major side-effects can occur in several organ systems, including:

1. GI tract;
2. kidney;
3. central nervous system;
4. liver;
5. respiratory system;
6. skin;
7. haematological reactions can also occur.

1. The GI System

The GI tract is the system most commonly affected by NSAIDs, which often leads to the discontinuation of treatment. Patients can experience:

- dyspepsia;
- epigastric pain;
- indigestion;
- nausea and vomiting.

GI effects may range from hyperaemia to diffuse gastritis, erosions or ulcers. Factors associated with increased risk of ulceration include:

- age (over 65 years);
- previous peptic ulcer disease;
- concomitant steroid therapy;
- heart failure;
- high-dose NSAIDs.

The use of NSAIDs in patients who have had a peptic ulcer is largely contraindicated. However, a patient with a history of gastric symptoms, such as indigestion, may be prescribed an NSAID with gastric cytoprotection. This includes H2 receptor antagonists for duodenal ulcers, for example cimetidine, and prostaglandin analogues for patients with gastric ulceration.

Proton pump inhibitors may also be considered. Drugs such as omeprazole and lansoprazole work by blocking the hydrogen–potassium adenosine triphosphatase enzyme system (the proton pump) of the gastric parietal cell, thereby inhibiting gastric acid production. They are effective in both the short- and long-term treatment of gastric and duodenal ulcers.

2. The Renal System

Patients at risk from NSAID renal insufficiency include those:

- with congestive heart failure;
- with cirrhosis and ascites;
- with nephrotic syndrome;
- over the age of 60;
- receiving concurrent diuretic therapy (which causes potassium retention).

Renal side-effects appear to be dose related and occur more frequently in the older population (Thompson and Dunne, 1995). NSAIDs also affect salt and water balance, which can cause hypertension and oedema in certain individuals. Acute interstitial nephritis and nephrotic syndrome can also occur.

3. The Central Nervous System

Early morning headache and dizziness can occur with indomethacin. Memory loss, inability to concentrate and cognitive dysfunction have been reported in older people following NSAID use (Goodwin and Regan, 1982).

4. The Liver

NSAID administration can cause a transient rise in liver enzymes. Those most at risk include older patients, individuals with poor renal function and patients taking a high dose of NSAIDs.

5. The Respiratory System

NSAIDs can cause the inhibition of cyclo-oxygenase in patients with bronchial asthma, precipitating bronchospasm. Asthma attacks can also occur in predisposed individuals.

6. The Skin

All NSAIDs can provoke skin reactions including photosensitivity, vesiculobullous, eruptions, urticaria, serum sickness and exfoliative erythroderma.

7. Haematological Reactions

The most common reaction is iron deficiency as a result of GI blood loss resulting from erosion or ulceration. NSAIDs can cause inhibition of platelet aggregation, prolonging bleeding time in patients. Blood dyscrasias are rare but among the major cause of death with this treatment. Agranulocytosis, thrombocytopenia, neutropenia and aplastic anaemia have all been reported.

Q3.15: Do NSAIDs interact with other medications?

NSAIDs do interact with a wide range of other treatments. For safe practice consult the manufacturers' guidelines before advocating use.

Q3.16: Are NSAIDs safe in pregnancy?

NSAIDs should be avoided during pregnancy, especially as they may promote premature closure of the ductus arteriosis and impair fetal circulation. They can also prolong gestation and increase post-partum and neonatal bleeding due to the inhibition of prostaglandin synthesis. Research is continuing on the effects of NSAIDs on infertility (Akil et al., 1996).

Section 3: Corticosteroids

Q3.17: What are corticosteroids?

Corticosteriods are synthetic derivatives of the body's naturally occurring corticosteroid hormones. The principal corticosteroid is cortisol, which is produced by the cortex of the adrenal glands, and its production is regulated by the hypothalamus and the pituitary gland via a negative feedback system.

Glucocorticoids are responsible for:

* carbohydrate, protein and fat metabolism;
* maintenance of blood sugar levels;
* the body's response to both physical and psychological stress;

- suppression of inflammation and the immune response (Christiansen and Krane, 1993).

Q3.18: In which conditions are corticosteroids used?

The role of steroids in the treatment of rheumatological conditions remains controversial because, whilst they are effective anti-inflammatory and immunosuppressive agents, they are also associated with potential serious side-effects. Corticosteroids have been used in the treatment of RA, often on a short-term basis to reduce increased disease activity.

Corticosteroids have been shown to be better than placebo and NSAIDs in the relief of pain and stiffness (George and Kirwan, 1990).

Corticosteroids are also used in the management of temporal arteritis, polymyalgia rheumatica, dermatomyositis, lupus erythematosus and in acute or life-threatening situations.

Q3.19: What dose of corticosteroids should be used in the treatment of rheumatological conditions?

Many factors will influence the dosage of steroids to be used in each individual patient including:

- the nature of the condition;
- the severity of the condition;
- clinical response.

Kirwan (1994) suggested the following treatment regime:

- low daily doses (up to 15 mg) to treat polymyalgia rheumatica and symptomatic RA;
- high daily doses (20–60 mg) for serious conditions, such as temporal arteritis;
- very high doses (intravenous) for acute or life-threatening situations.

Q3.20: How would you reduce the dose of corticosteroid in a patient with RA?

The exact method of reduction will depend on the clinical situation. Once the patient has shown signs of disease control by a reduction of symptoms and inflammatory blood parameters the dose of steroid can be decreased. The dose is often reduced slowly, sometimes by as little as 2.5 mg over one to two months. This rate of reduction is to try and prevent the patient experiencing corticosteroid withdrawal syndrome, which can occur as treatment is decreased. This syndrome can cause the patient to experience myalgia, fatigue and nausea, and has been reported in as many as 70% of patients treated with 30 mg prednisolone daily for longer than three months (Dixon and Christy, 1980).

Q3.21: Patients are often given a steroid card; why is this?

Patients are given a steroid card recording the dose and duration of their steroid treatment for their own safety. The administration of corticosteriods may result in the body's suppression of its own steroid production. If a patient was involved in an accident this could affect the immune response and would influence care management. Patients must be told not to stop taking their steroids unless under medical guidance as this action could lead to a complete halt of cortisol production, resulting in hypotension, hypoglycaemia and electrolyte imbalance.

Q3.22: What are the side-effects of corticosteriods?

Steroids can cause minor and major side-effects on most body organs. The potential side-effects are shown in Table 3.5.

Q3.23: How are corticosteroids administered?

Corticosteroids can be administered in a number of ways. These include oral, intravenous, IM, intra-articular (IA; into a joint) and into the soft tissue.

Table 3.5 Side-effects of corticosteriods

System	Side-effect	Comment
Metabolic	Obesity	Changes due to fat redistribution result in Cushingoid features such as Moon face
	Glucose/protein metabolism	Hyperglycaemia and insulin resistance occurs
	Hepatic enzyme induction	
Decreased resistance to infection		Due to immunosuppression. *Candida* and *Herpes zoster* infection has occurred in patients taking corticosteroids, along with a variety of bacterial infections
Musculoskeletal	Muscle wastage Tendon rupture	Due to protein catabolism Tendon rupture occurs with direct injection into tendon
	Osteoporosis	Occurs due to a reduction in calcium absorption into the bones and increase in calcium excretion. Vertebral wedge and crush fractures are a frequent complication of treatment
	Corticosteriod withdrawal syndrome	Occurs with long-term use of steroids (more than 7 days) and as a result of too rapid withdrawal. Symptoms include: myalgia, fatigue, malaise, anorexia, nausea, weight loss. Recommend a slow withdrawal appropriate to the length of time a patient has been on the steroid
GI	Peptic ulceration	Due to the inhibition of gastric prostaglandins which maintain the integrity of the gastric mucosa
	Pancreatitis	
Ophthalmic	Cataracts	
	Glaucoma	
Central nervous system	Psychosis	A paranoid and suicidal state may be induced by steroids
	Euphoria	
	Depression	
Skin	Acne	
	Striae	Due to protein catabolism. A symptom of Cushingoid side-effects
	Alopecia	
	Bruising	
	Skin atrophy	Due to protein catabolism
Growth retardation		
Adrenal suppression		

Oral

Enteric-coated tablets should always be prescribed to minimize gastric irritation, and always be administered with food. They are often prescribed on a daily or alternate day basis. Steroids should not be stopped without medical guidance.

Intravenous (Pulsed) Corticosteroids

There are many different treatment regimes but most include the administration of high-dose corticosteroid, usually 500 mg–1 g methylprednisolone over 30–60 minutes. The administration occurs on alternate days until three pulses have been given followed by a resting phase of about six weeks.

It can be used to reduce disease activity in conjunction with the commencement of suppressive drug therapy or, if the patient is experiencing a flare of symptoms, to induce remission. Methlyprednisolone has few side-effects (Weusten et al., 1993). Patients who experienced problems had compromised cardiovascular and immune systems as a result of their arthritis or concomitant drug therapy (Kirwan, 1995).

IM Corticosteroids

These are usually administered if the patient is experiencing an increase in the symptoms of his/her arthritis. It is important to give the injection deep into the muscle to prevent muscular atrophy occurring. Choy et al. (1993) found IM methylprednisolone was superior to equivalent oral doses of steroids.

IA Soft Tissue Injections

These are used to treat inflammation at specific sites, such as the knee or sub-acromial bursa. Patients should be advised to rest the injected joint for approximately 48 hours post injection to achieve the most beneficial effect. Any sign of heat or redness associated with increased pain following this period should be reported as this could be a sign of an infected joint. In comparison with oral steroids they are well tolerated and safe if administered properly. The Royal College of Nursing (RCN) Rheumatology Forum has produced guidelines on the administration of IA injections (see Q7.5).

Q3.24: What are corticosteroid-sparing agents?

This term is used to describe drugs which are prescribed to make it easier to reduce the dose of the steroid whilst at the same time controlling the underlying disease. Drugs such as azathioprine are used for this purpose.

Section 4: Disease-modifying Anti-rheumatic Drugs (DMARDs)

Q3.25: What are DMARDs?

DMARDs are prescribed in patients with inflammatory arthritis to suppress disease activity. They are also referred to as slow-acting anti-rheumatic drugs (SAARDs) or second-line agents. They are used in patients whose condition is active both clinically, when the patient experiences early morning stiffness and swollen joints for example, and on blood parameters, such as raised erythrocyte sedimentation rate (ESR) and C-reactive protein (CRP) (see Q2.34). Although DMARDs differ in their chemical composition they all possess common properties which include:

- delayed action: a therapeutic response takes three to six months to occur;
- their exact mode of action is poorly understood;
- their primary function is to suppress disease activity;
- all have the potential to cause adverse effects;
- the need for safety monitoring;

Current DMARDs in use are shown in Table 3.6.

Q3.26: What are the safety requirements for patients receiving DMARDs?

Most patients receiving DMARDs and cytotoxic agents require weekly blood tests for the first month of treatment and then usually at monthly intervals. These medications can cause bone marrow suppression, resulting in a reduction of red and white blood cells as well as affecting liver and kidney functions (this is discussed further in the section on investigation).

Table 3.6 DMARDs

Hydroxychloroquine/chloroquine
Dapsone
Sulphasalazine
Gold injections
Auranofin
D-penicillamine
Cyclosporin
Minocycline
Azathioprine
Methotrexate
Cyclophosphamide

Drugs such as gold and D-penicillamine will also require regular urinalysis. Different rheumatology units use different policies for monitoring drug therapy. There has been an attempt to standardize practice with the publication of guidelines from the British Society for Rheumatology but most units appear to adhere to their own policies based on their own experience of treatment. Kay and Puller (1992) found marked variation amongst respondents in monitoring schedules and interpretation of results. For legal implications it is necessary to be familiar with the data sheet recommendations. Table 3.7 shows the current monitoring regime in operation at the Staffordshire Rheumatology Centre.

Q3.27: What is gold (Myocrisin) therapy?

Gold is used as a long-term treatment for inflammatory joint disease (most commonly RA). Initially most patients are given a test dose of 10 mg IM and if no adverse effects are experienced progress to 50 mg IM weekly, reducing to 50 mg fortnightly as the patient responds, normally at around six months. With adequate control, frequency is reduced to monthly (around 12 months) and continued indefinitely unless side-effects occur.

Q3.28: What are the side-effects of gold therapy?

Toxicity is common with injectable gold, occurring in 30–40% of patients (Day, 1994). The nurse must be alert for a variety of reactions. These include the following.

Nephrotoxity

It is the responsibility of the nurse administering the injection of gold to test the urine prior to giving the injection. The RCN Rheumatology Forum has produced guidelines on the nurse's role in gold therapy (see Q7.3). Minor transient proteinuria is common but increasing proteinuria is an indication to stop gold. Treatment should be discontinued if a 24-hour protein urinalysis exceeds 1 g. Recovery is usual when gold is stopped. Isolated haematuria is not usually attributed to gold (Leonard et al., 1987).

Table 3.7 Monitoring regime for DMARDs at the Staffordshire Rheumatology Centre

Drug	Generic requirement	Specific requirement
(1) Sulphasalazine	FBC ESR	(1) Weekly LFTs for the first month, then monthly for six months and then twice yearly
	Platelets Differentials weekly for the first month and then monthly	
(2) Gold injections Auranofin D-penicillamine	"	(2) Weekly urinalysis
(3) Cyclosporin	"	(3) Creatinine, B/P weekly for one month, then monthly
(4) Methotrexate	"	(4) Weekly LFTs for the first month, then monthly
(5) Azathioprine	"	—
(6) Phenylbutazone	"	—
(7) Cyclophosphamide	"	(7)Weekly U&Es for the first month, then two to four weeks
(8) Dapsone	—	(8)Haemoglobin after first week

Key: BP — blood pressure
ESR – erythrocyte sedimentation rate
FBC – full blood count
LFT – liver function tests

Skin Reactions

Minor rashes and pruritus can be treated symptomatically with aqueous cream or 0.5% hydrocortisone cream. Mouth ulcers occur less often than a rash. Gold should be withheld if there is widespread pruritus, severe or rapidly progressive rash or stomatitis, as these can be associated with exfoliative dermatitis.

Pulmonary Reactions

Hypersensitivity pneumonitis, which is distinguishable from rheumatoid lung owing to its acute onset, will necessitate the discontinuation of gold therapy.

Vasomotor Reactions

These are often referred to as 'nitroid' reactions, which may occur within minutes of administration and necessitate the patient remaining in a clinic for a period of time following the injection. Reactions are characterized by weakness, nausea, sweating, facial flushing, erythema and hypotension.

Post-injection Reactions

The patient may experience transient polyarthralgia, myalgia, joint swelling, fatigue and malaise. It can be difficult at times to distinguish these effects from the symptoms of active inflammatory disease.

Haematological

A rapid or progressive downward trend in neutrophils, sometimes accompanied by a fall in platelets, can be an indication of bone marrow suppression. Thrombocytopenia will occur in 1–3% of patients receiving IM gold. This can be serious and require treatment with corticosteroids.

Q3.29: How is oral gold different from IM gold?

Oral gold (Auranofin) has a completely different chemical structure from injectable gold and is less potent. Diarrhoea is often the commonest side-effect and may respond to the introduction of bulking agents such as bran or a temporary reduction in dosage. It requires the same surveillance as IM gold.

Q3.30: When is D-penicillamine (Distamine) used?

D-penicillamine is used in the treatment of RA and scleroderma. Dosages commence at 125 mg daily and can be increased to 750 mg/1000 mg daily to obtain disease control. The incidence of toxicity increases as the dose increases (Kay, 1986). Tablets should be taken on an empty stomach and not with iron tablets or milk, which would impair the drug absorption.

Q3.31: What are the side-effects of D-penicillamine?

d-Penicillamine possesses the same potential haematological and urinary side-effects as gold therapy. Minor rashes can be treated symptomatically but severe rashes are the most worrying and would lead to the discontinuation of treatment. Patients who have a penicillin allergy are at greatest risk of experiencing a mucocutaneous reaction. Patients may also experience an alteration in taste sensation. Myasthenia gravis is a rare complication that can occur after years of uneventful therapy and take over a year to resolve.

Q3.32: For what conditions is sulphasalazine used?

Sulphasalazine is used in the treatment of RA, spondyloarthropathies and reactive arthritis. It is the most popular first choice of DMARD amongst rheumatologists (Kay and Puller, 1992). To reduce the likelihood of nausea the drug is usually commenced at 500 mg daily increasing by 500 mg at weekly intervals to the usual maintenance dose of 1 g twice daily. An enteric-coated preparation is used to reduce the likelihood of GI symptoms.

Q3.33: What are the side-effects of sulphasalazine?

Only 20–25% of patients will need to stop treatment because of toxicity (Amos et al., 1986). The commonest side-effects occur on the GI and central nervous systems, and include nausea, vomiting, anorexia, dyspepsia, light-headedness and dizziness. If a patient experiences any of these symptoms the dose should be reduced to the previously tolerated level and any further increases should be attempted at a slower rate. Skin rashes will occur in 5% of patients taking sulphasalazine (Amos et al., 1986). If the rash occurs within the first 14 days of treatment a desensitization programme can be tried. Initially given in 1 mg doses, sulphasalazine is built up over 25–56 days. Successful desensitization has been achieved in 85% of patients with RA (Amos et al., 1986).

Haematological reactions can include leucopenia. This is most likely to occur in the first six months of treatment, although it can occur at any time. It is the commonest potential serious side-effect associated with this drug. Thrombocytopenia occurs less frequently.

Allergic hepatic reactions and hepatitis can occur, necessitating discontinuation of therapy. LFTs must be carried out as part of the monitoring requirements.

Q3.34: When are cytotoxic agents used in rheumatology?

Methotrexate (MTX), azathioprine and cyclophosphamide are all agents used in the treatment of rheumatological conditions. Cyclophosphamide is a strong drug that is used to achieve immuno-suppression in systemic lupus erythematosus, vasculitis, resistant rheumatic arthritis, polyarteritis nodosa, Wegner's granulomatosis and myositis. It requires careful hospital monitoring.

MTX is the most commonly used cytotoxic drug. It is given weekly either orally or IM in doses between 5 mg and 25 mg. The RCN Rheumatology Forum has produced guidelines for nurses involved in the administration of IM MTX (see Q7.4). Folic acid is often prescribed with MTX to reduce the likelihood of minor side-effects occurring, such as stomatitis. A chest X-ray is taken prior to the commencement of treatment, as pre-existing lung disease requires special attention. Alcohol should be avoided. Trimethoprin and co-trimoxazole (e.g. Septrin and Bactrim) should not be prescribed in patients taking MTX because of their anti-folate action.

Q3.35: What are side-effects of MTX therapy?

Common side-effects include nausea and vomiting and may necessi-tate anti-emetic treatment on the day of MTX administration and for the following 24–48 hours. If nausea is a problem and doubts about absorption exist then the drug can be given IM.

Leucopenia is the most common bone marrow toxicity (Kremer

and Joong, 1986). Hepatotoxicity, defined as elevation of transaminase, can occur and MTX should be stopped if there is a persistent elevation of this marker.

Acute pneumonitis is potentially serious and should be considered if there is a dry cough and recent breathlessness.

Q3.36: What haematological and biochemical levels would necessitate discontinuation of DMARDs and cytotoxic agents?

Medications should be stopped if the following levels are reported:

- total white cell count $< 3 \times 10^9/l$;
- neutrophils $< 2 \times 10^9/l$;
- platelets $< 120 \times 10^9/l$;
- deteriorating liver function.

Q3.37: What other disease-modifying agents are used in the management of rheumatological conditions?

Cyclosporin (Neoral) is used in RA, Behçet's disease and other cell-mediated chronic inflammatory conditions. Nephrotoxicity can occur and is dose related. Serum creatinine and blood pressure require attention.

Hydroxychloroquine and chloroquine are used in patients with less aggressive RA. These medications do not require blood monitoring but an eye examination should be carried out on a yearly basis to detect retinal alterations.

Phenylbutazone is available only on hospital prescription for patients with ankylosing spondylitis and other spondylo-arthropathies. Phenylbutazone is an NSAID that may also affect the immune response (Furst, 1988). Blood monitoring is required with this medication.

Minocycline is a broad-spectrum antibiotic often prescribed in the treatment of acne but also used in patients with RA. Blood monitoring is required; this includes FBC and LFTs.

Q3.38: Can patients on DMARDs have vaccinations?

Live vaccines include:
- measles;

- rubella;
- BCG;
- mumps;
- poliomyelitis;
- yellow fever;
- typhoid (oral).

These should be avoided in patients taking azathioprine, MTX, cyclophosphamide and high doses of corticosteroids. Patients on these medications should avoid contact with people who have chickenpox or *Herpes zoster* infection. If they experience these conditions they may require varicella zoster immunoglobulin, administered in the hospital setting. In general vaccination is safe for patients taking gold, d-penicillamine and sulphasalazine although it is still preferable to avoid live vaccines.

Q3.39: Are DMARDs safe during pregnancy?

Women with RA often need to achieve disease suppression to increase their chance of conceiving. Decisions regarding the withdrawal of potentially toxic drug therapy need to be made in good time since many drugs can affect the vulnerable stages of embryogenesis. Teratogenic agents should be discontinued at least six months before attempting conception. These include MTX, azathioprine and cyclophosphamide. The effects of rheumatological drug therapy in pregnancy are shown are Table 3.8.

Case Study

Jenny is 34 years of age. For the past two months she has been experiencing pain and stiffness in her hands and feet. Her GP prescribed an NSAID (diclofenac 75mg bd), which helped initially, but now Jenny is finding it ineffective in reducing the pain and stiffness. The GP referred Jenny to a rheumatologist. Clinical examination and investigations revealed:

- *bilateral synovitis in the hands and feet;*
- *small effusion in the right knee;*
- *early morning stiffness lasting for over two hours;*

- *haematological and biochemical evidence of disease activity, e.g. ESR 40 mm/h, CRP 85 mg/100ml;*
- *X-ray evidence of soft tissue swelling and peri-articular osteopenia.*

A diagnosis of RA is confirmed and Jenny is commenced on sulphasalazine (a DMARD). Jenny finds that after three months of taking this her symptoms settle down and she begins to feel well in herself again. She continues with this treatment for three years, before encountering a severe increase in the pain, stiffness and fatigue. Investigations at this time reveal a further increase in the activity of the arthritis, with the presence of a positive rheumatoid factor. X-rays of the hands also show evidence of erosion. It is clear that the sulphasalazine is no longer being effective and the presence of erosions necessitates the need for stronger drug therapy to regain control of the condition. Jenny is commenced on MTX and after a few months finds that her symptoms are greatly reduced. It is important that Jenny and all patients with RA are reviewed regularly to assess the efficacy of their present drug treatment.

Table 3.8 Drugs and pregnancy

Drug	Effect on pregnancy
(1) Analgesia	Paracetamol can be taken during pregnancy
(2) NSAIDs	May lead to premature closure of the ductus arteriosus Aspirin can cause cleft palate Avoid during late pregnancy; may cause prolonged gestation and labour and increased blood loss at delivery antepartum haemorrhage.
(3) Corticosteroids	Considered safe when taken in low dosages (5–10 mg daily). If withdrawn within two months of labour steroid cover should be provided
(4) DMARDs	
Gold and D-penicillamine	Effects during pregnancy are not known
Auranofin	A number of patients have been treated throughout their pregnancies with auranofin; all gave birth to healthy infants
Sulphasalazine	Avoid in late pregnancy – neonatal jaundice
Anti-malarials	Not recommended; may cause congenital deafness
(5) Cytotoxic medications	All teratogenic

Section 5: Investigations

Q3.40: What investigations are carried out in relation to drug therapy?

A full blood count (FBC) will identify some key side-effects from treatment.

- *Haemoglobin*: The typical anaemia of RA is a normocytic, normochromic anaemia with a haemoglobin of around 10–12 g/dl. The cause of anaemia is multifactorial. Iron utilization is impaired and there is a correlation between disease activity and the severity of the anaemia. Bone marrow suppression secondary to drug treatment can cause anaemia and NSAIDs can cause intestinal blood loss. The mechanism of sulphasalazine and MTX can cause a macrocytic macrochromic anaemia.
- *Leucocytes*: There are five different types of leucocytes. An FBC measures both the collective number and the individual number of cells. Leucocytes include:
  - (a) monocytes: these cells play a key role as antigen-presenting cells;
  - (b) basophils: these mature in the tissues, becoming mast cells, and release histamine and small quantities of bradykinin and serotonin during inflammation;
  - (c) eosinophils: these are involved in the pathogenesis of hyper-sensitivity. Numbers are greatly increased in the blood during an allergic reaction. Eosinophilia can be associated with a rash during gold therapy;
  - (d) neutrophils: these cells attack bacterial invasion and make up 40–75% of total white blood cells;
  - (e) lymphocytes: there are two types of lymphocytes. B lympho-cytes produce antibodies and T lymphocytes are responsible for the elimination of viruses and other microorganisms that infect the cell of the host. A normal immune response requires adequate numbers of both types of lymphocytes.
- *Platelets*: A raised number of platelets (thrombocytosis) can occur in active RA and may correlate with the number of joints involved and the amount of active synovitis. A reduced platelet count (thrombocytopenia) is rare in RA except when it is related to DMARDs.

Q.3.41: What factors can cause a low white blood cell count (leucopenia)?

A low white blood cell count will reduce the body's protection against infection. If the neutrophil count falls below $0.5 \times 10^9/l$ patients are likely to become susceptible to frequently recurring bacterial infections. Causes of leucopenia include:

- Felty's syndrome;
- aplastic anaemia;
- systemic lupus erythematosus;
- side-effects of DMARDs;
- acquired immune deficiency syndrome;
- Hodgkin's disease.

Q3.42: What is the purpose of individual biochemical investigations?

(a) Liver function abnormalities may be a result of:

- an active inflammatory condition such as RA;
- side-effects of medications such as MTX, sulphasalazine and NSAIDs;
- Felty's syndrome. Liver involvement may be present in up to 65% of patients with Felty's syndrome.

(b) Kidney function abnormalities may result from:

- glomerulitis vasculitis
- amyloidosis
- drugs such as gold, d-penicillamine, cyclosporin and NSAIDs. Renal involvement caused by nephrotoxic drugs is most likely to be seen first on routine urine testing.

Q3.43: What factors should be noted on urine testing?

Urinalysis is a valuable tool in the surveillance of drug therapy, especially in terms of toxicity.

- *Appearance:* Sulphasalazine can cause orange discolouration. Patients need to know that this is a normal feature of the medication.

- *Odour:* Infected urine has a characteristic 'fishy' smell. Sulphasalazine and d-penicillamine also have their own specific odours.
- *Glucose:* This is not usually present in the urine. In a patient on corticosteroids it raises the possibility of drug-induced diabetes mellitus.
- *Blood:* The presence of blood is often found to be of no significance but requires investigation if it is a persistent finding. Haematuria can be an early indication of polyarteritis and 50% of patients with lupus will have small amounts of blood and protein in their urine. The patient should be referred if haematuria persists over a six-month period. The presence of more than 100 red cells in a midstream specimen necessitates an early referral.
- *Protein:* The presence of protein in the urine can indicate:
  - infection: this will require treatment to prevent a flare of disease activity;
  - amyloid disease;
  - nephropathy due to gold or D-penicillamine;
  - glomerular dysfunction in conditions such as lupus.

The Use of Drug Therapy in other Rheumatological Conditions

Q3.44: How is gout managed pharmacologically?

The drug management of gout occurs in two stages:

1. the reduction of inflammatory joint symptoms;
2. the long-term management of persistent hyperuricaemia.

The Reduction of Inflammatory Joint Symptoms

NSAIDs are used in the management of acute episodes of gout. The NSAID prescribed will be influenced by the patient's tolerance and the clinician's choice. Although many NSAIDs have been found to be equally efficacious, indomethacin is still often regarded as the drug of choice. Complete resolution of inflammation can require anything between two days and two weeks of treatment.

When NSAIDs are contraindicated (see Table 3.4), colchicine is prescribed. This is usually administered in a dose of 1 mg followed by increases of 0.5 mg every two hours until symptoms settle or GI symptoms occur. The maximum dose of colchicine is 10 mg.

Long-term Management of Gout

Regular drug therapy will be required if there are:

- visible tophi and/or erosions revealed by radiological examinations;
- renal impairment;
- recurrent attacks of acute gout.

The choice of agents includes:

- uricosuric drugs, e.g. probenecid or sulphinpyrazone;
- a xanthine-oxidase inhibitor e.g. allopurinol.

Both groups require co-administration of an NSAID or colchicine for at least the first four months of treatment because hypouricaemic drugs increase the risk of acute attacks of gout during the first few months of therapy.

> **Q3.45: What drugs are used in the management of established osteoporosis?**

There are several drugs used to treat osteoporosis; choice may depend on the individual patient's requirements and on the clinician's preference.

1. Hormone Replacement Therapy (HRT)

It has been reported that HRT prevents bone loss and fracture in post-menopausal women (Snaith, 1996). To reduce the risk of fracture HRT should be started soon after the menopause and be taken for 10 years. Women should be offered advice concerning the current research findings on benefits and side-effects of HRT.

2. Bisphosphonates

These drugs coat the bone surface, making them less susceptible to osteoclastic activity.

- *Cyclical etidronate therapy (Didronel PMO):* This treatment comprises a 14-day course of disodium etidronate 400 mg daily. It should be taken at least two hours after one meal and two hours before the next meal (e.g. at the midpoint of a four-hour fast) to aid its poor absorption. After the 14-day course, the individual would commence 500 mg elemental calcium for 76 days. Studies have shown an increase in bone density and a reduction in the incidence of vertebral fractures with this therapy (Storm et al., 1990).

- *Alendronate (Fosamax):* This medication is taken as a single 10 mg daily dose, on an empty stomach. It needs to be administered 30 minutes before breakfast and it must be taken with a full glass of plain tap water. It is recommended that the patient does not lie down after taking this drug, to minimize the risk of upper GI irritation. There is evidence that this preparation increases bone density and reduces the risk of new vertebral fractures occurring (Recker et al., 1995).

Bisphosphonates have few side-effects, although nausea, dyspepsia and diarrhoea have all been reported. Alendronate should be used with caution in women with existing upper GI problems. This treatment is often prescribed for the older woman with established osteoporosis who does not wish to use HRT. It can also be used in men with osteoporosis although there is a lack of research data to support its efficacy.

3. Calcium Supplements

These decrease bone loss but not to the same extent as other anti-resorptive agents.

4. Calcitonin

This potent agent has a rapid but short-lived effect on osteoblast function. Side-effects include nausea and vomiting, diarrhoea, dizziness and headache, which may be reduced by intranasal administration.

5. Vitamin D

This vitamin is required to absorb calcium. It may be appropriate to use this supplementation in the house-bound older person who may well have a reduced intake of Vitamin D. A study in a French nursing home revealed that the administration of calcium and vitamin D reduced the risk of hip fracture by 43% (Chapuy et al., 1992).

6. Vitamin D Metabolites

People with established osteoporosis have lower calcium absorption than age-matched controls. This can be addressed by giving low doses of vitamin D metabolites, including calcitriol and alfacalcidol.

7. Anabolic Agents

These agents stimulate bone formation and include sodium fluoride and parathyroid hormone. Their current use is experimental and they are not licensed for the treatment of osteoporosis in the UK.

> **Q3.46: Is it useful to check blood calcium levels, and if so how often should they be checked?**

There is no benefit in checking blood calcium levels.

Conclusion

Drug therapy is an important aspect of the care management of many rheumatology conditions, especially RA. The nurse must be able to discuss the role of drug interventions with the patient and the family, thereby enabling the patient to become an active recipient of care. If drug therapy can minimize pain, stiffness and disease activity then it is a useful adjunct to other interventions.

Chapter 4
Patient Education

In the rheumatic diseases, self-care activities and self-management play a pivotal role in attaining an efficacious outcome, and patient education (PE) is the method used to equip patients to undertake these tasks. Many rheumatic diseases such as osteoarthritis (OA) and rheumatoid arthritis (RA) are chronic and incurable and have an unpredictable day-to-day pattern of activity, and so patients need to be able to tailor their drugs and treatments accordingly (Hill, 1995). To enable them to do this they will require:

1. the knowledge to self-manage their condition;
2. confidence in their ability to make a positive difference.

A partnership approach to disease management between the practitioner and patient serves to empower the patient, and if he/she is in part responsible for the choice of treatment, be it exercise or drug therapy, this will encourage him/her to adhere to it (see Q2.9). PE is not merely the transfer of knowledge from nurse to the patient; this is defined as patient teaching (Lorig, 1996). In addition to the acquisition of information, PE involves persuading patients to adopt beneficial behaviours and to achieve positive attitudes. A simple working definition modified from Lorig (1996) is: 'Any set of planned educational activities designed to improve the patient's health behaviours and through this their health status and ultimately their long term outcome' (Hill 1997a).

PE is based on self-efficacy theory. Self-efficacy refers to the person's confidence in his/her ability to perform a specific task or achieve a particular objective (Bandura, 1977). Increases in self-efficacy are thought to bring about increases in appropriate health behaviours and health outcomes.

Q4.2: What are the aims of PE?

The aim of any PE programme is to improve the patient's health status, which will ultimately lead to a better health outcome. For some rheumatology patients this aim is unobtainable, and in these cases preservation of the status quo or slowing of deterioration is a reasonable alternative. Whatever the eventual outcome of the disease process, the quality of life throughout the illness journey will have been improved with PE.

It is important when working in a collaborative health professional/patient partnership that each knows the boundaries of their responsibilities:

- The primary responsibility for the overall management of the disease remains with health professionals.
- The day-to-day control of illness and symptoms is the remit of the patient.

If patients are to undertake this role successfully they will have to learn to:

- vary drug usage according to their symptoms;
- tailor their daily exercise routine;
- employ coping techniques;
- plan periods of activity/rest.

A PE programme needs to be designed to fulfil these requirements, whatever disease the patient has.

Q4.3: Is PE effective?

The first question that should be asked is, 'What do we mean by effectiveness?'. Two definitions that are particularly relevant are:

1. PE can be considered to be an effective therapy if it brings benefits over and above the existing treatments (Hill, 1997a). A review of the literature of 45 studies undertaken between 1987 and 1991

showed that when PE was added to existing treatments patients improved by 15–30% (Hirano et al., 1994).

2. PE should achieve benefits comparable to those resulting from conventional therapy but with fewer side-effects or at a lower cost (DeVellis and Blalock, 1993).

The research undertaken to date has shown PE to be effective in a number of areas (Table 4.1).

Table 4.1 The effects of PE

Domain	Specific outcome
Knowledge	Increases in knowledge of: disease process drugs exercise joint protection
Behaviour	Increases in practice of: exercise joint protection relaxation
Health status	Reduction in levels of: anxiety depression pain disability

Q4.4: What should be included in a PE programme?

Each patient is an individual and needs to acquire different information. However, there is patient concurrence on some topics. For instance, the Arthritis Research Campaign (ARC) report that nearly all patients questioned in one study said they wanted an honest and balanced view of their condition that includes a full package of information. The information should be:

• up to date;
• provide reassurance;
• cover drugs and treatments;

- include self-management, diet and exercise, and give practical tips;
- help patients to communicate effectively with medical practitioners in the hospital and community setting.

Many nurse specialists (Hill et al., 1994) and some practice/district nurses (Dargie and Proctor, 1993) undertake PE programmes for rheumatology patients. The programmes are usually based on the major problems that patients encounter and the topics covered usually include those shown in Table 4.2.

Table 4.2 Content of a typical PE programme

Subject	Content
Knowledge of disease	Aetiology and symptoms
Drug treatments	Usage, effects, adverse effects
Pain control	Drugs, relaxation, distraction etc.
Exercise	How, what, and when?
Protecting joints	Reducing load, using splints
Controlling fatigue	Causes, conserving energy, enhancing sleep
Complementary therapy	Acupuncture, massage, aromatherapy
The effects of diet	Reducing weight, effects of health, fatigue
Coping strategies	Contracting, practical methods, self-efficacy
Surviving a flare	What it is and how to cope
The role of self-help	Effects of self-efficacy, voluntary organizations
Communicating	How to get the best out of health professionals
Goal setting	How to set achievable targets and reach them

It is important to document what topic has been covered and an example of a PE Checksheet is shown in Figure 4.1. Not all patients will need to cover all topics: this will be dependent on their existing knowledge and diagnosis. For instance, a patient with newly diagnosed acute gout will initially need information about:

- the disease and investigations;
- drug therapy;
- pain control;
- diet.

This may well suffice unless they experience a further attack. However, a patient with RA may need to experience the whole programme, particularly if his/her disease is unremitting.

PE Checksheet

Name: Diagnosis:
                                   Date Diagnosed:

Topic	Establish shared goals	Verbal Explanation	Written Information	Other	Date
Disease process/investigations					
Drug therapy					
Pain control					
Exercise					
Joint protection, splints, shoes etc.					
Controlling fatigue					
Complementary therapies					
Diet					
Coping strategies					
Managing a flare					
Self-help voluntary organisations					
Tips on communicating with HP's					
Goals set					

Figure 4.1 PE checklist; HPs = health professionals.

Q4.5: How can we assess prior knowledge and set shared goals?

All patients will have some knowledge of their disease, for instance they will all know that one of the prime symptoms is pain. They may also have some misinformation that can be detrimental to their health status. An example would be the common misconception that all people who have RA become disabled and there are also many misunderstandings about drug therapy (Hill et al., 1991). If patients are under the care of a rheumatologist they may have undertaken a PE programme at their local hospital. To assist in formulating the PE programme it is necessary to establish the patient's knowledge base. One reasonably quick and easy way of doing this is to give patients a questionnaire such as the Patient Knowledge Questionnaire (Hill et al., 1991) that they can complete at home and bring with them to their consultation. This is the method used for patients in general practice by Dargie and Proctor (1993).

Q4.6: Is assessment of patients' beliefs important?

One of the key aims of a PE programme is to bring about beneficial behaviour change and so it is important to discover what patients believe about their disease and treatments. For instance, patients may not wish to undertake an exercise programme because they believe that the increased pain incurred means they have damaged their joints or they may refuse an intra-articular injection of steroid because they believe that steroids will cause them to 'put on weight'. The best way to find out their beliefs is to ask open-ended questions such as 'Why don't you exercise every day?' or 'What do you think will happen if you have a steroid injection?'. Beliefs can be very difficult to alter, particularly if they are an inherent part of the patient's culture, and it is best not to interfere unless the belief is detrimental to his/her health.

Q4.7: Which is the best way to deliver a PE programme?

There are a number of ways to deliver a PE programme (Table 4.3) and each has its merits.

Table 4.3 Methods of delivering a PE programme

Mode of delivery	Method	Educator
One to one	Individual teaching	Nurse
Opportunity education	Individual teaching	Nurse
Groups	Group teaching	Nurse/health professional
Arthritis self-management group	Group teaching	Lay person/health professional

Individual PE

In general practice PE is usually undertaken on a one-to-one basis. This is the most flexible format as the PE programme can be tailored to each individual. Some practices hold nurse-run arthritis clinics (Bird, 1993; Dickson, 1993) at which each intervention can be planned over a series of visits. If this is the case there will be time to:

- explore the patient's needs;
- make an in-depth assessment of his/her knowledge;
- establish shared goals;
- discuss the preferred method of transfer of information.

Opportunity Education

Even in practices where there is no planned provision for PE, there is opportunity to educate. Patients with RA may be attending the nurse for regular blood tests or intramuscular (IM) gold or methotrexate injections (see Chapter 3). These are ideal opportunities to discuss drug therapy and any problems arising from their disease. Likewise, patients on the elderly register may be experiencing problems arising from OA. Again this is a unique opportunity to undertake PE.

Other opportunities would be when patients attend for:

- flu injections: patients are often elderly and may have OA;
- cervical smears: any patient with RA, OA of the hip or ankylosing spondylitis could experience physical problems having sexual intercourse;
- hypertension clinics: patients, often elderly, may have OA and patients with gout may also have hypertension.

This type of short unplanned encounter is called 'opportunity education'.

Teaching in Groups

This is a very popular format as it can reach more patients in one session, is less labour intensive than individual PE and therefore cheaper. It is a useful method of transferring general information:

- facts about different forms of arthritis;
- an overview of different types of medication;
- methods of joint protection;
- relaxation techniques.

Group teaching is less useful for patients who:

- have difficulty learning;
- are going onto a specific drug therapy;
- require an individual exercise programme.

These patients will need to be seen in a one-to-one session.

When teaching patients in groups it is important to try to meet each participant's expectations, and there are three important aspects that need to be made clear at the outset:

1. what you expect to achieve during the course;
2. what is included in the programme;
3. who the programme is aimed at.

Group participation can be a very positive experience both medically and socially, and research has shown that patients do indeed learn from each other (Campbell et al., 1995).

Arthritis Self Management Programmes (ASMP)

The ASMP is a group programme that was developed in the USA by Lorig and colleagues (Lorig et al., 1985) and is based on self-efficacy theory. It has been shown to be remarkably effective and has been adapted for use in many countries including the UK. The topics taught are similar to those in other programmes but this one is based on the premise that effective PE requires behavioural changes to occur and so emphasis is placed on:

- problem-solving strategies;
- development of coping skills;
- management of symptoms;
- utilization of information.

There is also a further vital difference from other programmes: the people who teach. The courses are taught by a lay teacher who normally has some form of arthritis, and a health professional. The ASMP is community based and taught over a period of months in six two-hourly sessions. Further information regarding the ASMP can be obtained from Arthritis Care.

Learning Aids

Verbal information

There are a number of modalities that can enhance learning (Table 4.4); the most common technique is by verbal communication.

Table 4.4 Learning aids

Verbal information
Written information
Videos
Audiocassettes
Computer-assisted learning

Good communication skills will be further enhanced if the educator watches the patient carefully, taking cues as to when he/she is ready to receive the information. The effectiveness of the education also depends on it being given:

- at the right time;
- at the right speed;
- using appropriate lay language.

Verbal information may be misinterpreted and is easily forgotten; in fact most of us when visiting our general practitioner (GP) or outpatient clinic recall only about 40% of what we are told! Simple guidelines to aid memory retention are given in Table 4.5. It is best

Table 4.5 Guidelines for giving verbal information

Give the most important information first

- We remember best what we are told first

Give consideration to the patient's priorities

- It is easier to recall what we consider is most important

Do not bombard patients with too many facts at once

- We only remember the first four or five facts we are told

Provide written back-up

- This can be read and re-read at leisure

to back up verbal explanations with written information that can be taken home and read at leisure. Also remember to use the PE Check-sheet (Figure 4.1) to record what has been taught.

Written information

There is evidence that written information is effective (Hill et al., 1997), and research has shown that patients feel the need of it (Donovan and Blake, 1992). There is excellent written information available on a wide range of topics. The ARC and Arthritis Care produce booklets about specific diseases and treatments, and many pharmaceutical companies provide drug information leaflets (DILs) about their products which are intended for patients. However, it may be necessary to compile some patient information yourself. For instance, DILs are often produced in-house because prescribing and monitoring practice vary from area to area. It is very important that information is written in lay language at a level that is easily understood by the patients and a good example is shown in Figure 4.2.

Guidelines to writing user-friendly material are given in Table 4.6. Further information about readability and designing written material can be found in Hill (1998b).

Table 4.6 Guidelines for writing patient literature

Start with the aims of the material
Keep the sentence structure simple
Stick to one- or two-syllable words
Use a limited number of words using three or more syllables
Write in short sentences
Use short paragraphs
Use a question-and-answer format
Try not to use medical terminology, e.g. say knee cap rather than patella
Use positive rather than negative language
Make the material sound personal by using words such as I, we, us
Include information that the patients ask for as well as what they should know

Video

Written material, even when pitched at the easy-to-read level, may be unsuitable for those who have poor reading skills, are dyslexic or are partially sighted. Videos are a useful alternative and an excellent

What is methotrexate?

Methotrexate is one of a group of drugs know as disease-modifying drugs. It is used to treat several types of arthritis, including rheumatoid arthritis. It usually comes as a tablet but it can be given by injection.

How does it work?

It is thought to slow down disease activity. It can also make your immune system (your body's defence system) less effective and so it is always used with care. It is not a painkiller, and so you should continue taking your usual anti-inflammatory tablets and painkillers.

How long will it take to work?

Methotrexate builds up slowly in the body so it does not work straight away. You may start to feel better after only three weeks, but it could take 12 weeks or even longer.

What dose will I take?

When you first start on methotrexate you will begin on a very small dose. This will be increased slowly until you reach your normal dose as follows:

2.5 mg a week for one week
5.0 mg a week for one week
7.5 mg a week for one week
10 mg a week as your normal dose

A few people need a higher dose than 10 mg a week and it can be taken in doses up to 25 mg a week in some cases.

When should I take the tablets?

You will only take methotrexate once a week. You can take it at any time of the day but you should always try to take it on the same day each week. Because you only take it once a week it is easy to forget. Most people find it best to get into a routine of always taking it at the same time on the same day; before breakfast on Friday, for example.

Take methotrexate with a full glass of water on an *empty* stomach. If it gives you indigestion take it with a little food such as a cream cracker.

How long can I stay on the tablets?

If you have no bad side-effects you can stay on them for as long as they are helping. Some people have been taking them for many years.

Are there any side-effects?

Only a few people get side-effects. They usually occur when you first start taking the tablets. They are *usually mild* and get better in a few hours. They are:

Feeling sick	Diarrhoea	Headaches	Hair thinning
Indigestion	Skin rash	Mouth ulcers	

(contd)

More important side-effects are:
Large bruises caused by changes in the clotting cells (platelets) in the blood.
Sore throat and fever caused by changes in the white cells that fight infections.
Sudden breathlessness or cough.

What should I do if I get side-effects?
If you get side-effects tell the doctor or nurse *straight away*.

Do I need special tests because of my tablets?
Yes. Before you begin your methotrexate you should always have a chest X-ray. When you first start on methotrexate your blood must be tested every two weeks for the first eight weeks and then once a month. You will need these tests all the time that you are on the tablets, to check that your blood can clot properly and that your white cells can fight infection.

If your GP checks your blood, phone the surgery and ask if your blood tests are normal. If there are any problems you may have to stop taking the tablets for a while until your blood gets back to normal.

Can I take other medicines with my tablets?
Some medicines do not mix well with methotrexate and should not be taken with it.
They are:

* trimethoprim;
* sulphonamides;
* probenecid;
* phenylbutazone;
* some anti-inflammatory tablets including aspirin.

Always remind your doctor that you are taking methotrexate if he/she prescribes other medicines for you. You should always tell the chemist if you buy 'over-the-counter' medicine.

Is there anything else that I must be careful of?
If you have never had chickenpox and come into contact with someone who has chickenpox or shingles, you must tell your doctor immediately.

If you catch chickenpox or shingles tell your doctor immediately.

You should not have a vaccination that uses a 'live vaccine' (polio or German measles are the most common). Flu vaccines are safe. To be certain, tell the doctor or nurse that you are on methotrexate before you have a vaccination.

Avoid alcohol, but the occasional moderate drink on a special occasion will do you no harm.

Is methotrexate safe in pregnancy?
Methotrexate can harm an unborn baby. Do not use if you are pregnant. If you get pregnant while you are taking methotrexate, tell your doctor as soon as you know. If you are planning to have a baby, discuss it with your doctor or nurse. You should stop taking methotrexate six months before you plan to have a baby. This applies to men as well as women.

(contd)

You should not breast feed while you are on methotrexate.
Methotrexate can reduce sperm count in men.

Remember to keep all medicines out of the reach of children

Figure 4.2 Methotrexate information list.

method of demonstrating exercise regimes and joint-protection techniques. Again, the ARC and Arthritis Care produce videos.

Audiocassettes

Audiocassettes transform written information into a verbal format and are useful for patients who cannot read or have sight difficulties. They are easily transported and so can be used at any time on a portable machine. Many relaxation programmes are in this format but there is no reason why drug information or other PE modules cannot be transferred to tape.

Computer-assisted learning

Although at an earlier phase of development, computer technology has the potential to make vast inroads in PE. Expert systems are being developed that will provide a truly patient-centred approach as they allow patients to seek information at will and in any order they wish. All those who own a personal computer can have access to the Internet and it is becoming more commonplace for patients to search the Net for information about their disease and treatments. Perhaps the time will come when each surgery has a computer that patients can access whilst sitting waiting for their appointment.

Case Study

Wendy is a 59-year-old woman who has had a diagnosis of polyarthritis for 4 years. She is currently taking piroxicam 20 mg daily and co-proxamol as necessary. Over the last few months she has been experiencing a lot more pain in her hands and feet and it has also spread to involve both of her knees. She was seen by the GP who made a referral to the local rheumatologist, who confirmed that she had RA and added oral methotrexate (MTX) 10 mg weekly and folic acid to her drug regimen. Whilst at the hospital she was also seen by the clinical nurse specialist (CNS) who discussed her drug therapy and diagnosis. Unfortunately she experienced side-effects to the MTX, which was changed from the oral to IM version as this has a lower side-effect profile. The practice agreed to administer the MTX and monitor Joyce's progress.

She attended the practice nurse clinic to receive her MTX and have her bloods taken. At this point she was clearly concerned about her drug therapy and although the CNS has talked to her about the MTX and given her a DIL (Figure 4.2), she was confused about the different drugs she was taking and what they were for. The practice nurse gave her an information leaflet about drug therapy for RA and the purpose of the MTX, non-steroidal anti-inflammatory drugs and analgesics, together with a knowledge questionnaire (PKQ). A longer appointment was made to discuss her drug therapy further, and she was asked to bring her DIL along and to write down any queries or worries about her RA and its treatment.

When she returned to the practice, the PKQ highlighted that she was unable to differentiate between her drugs and she knew little about the importance of exercise and joint protection. During her consultation she asked many questions about her drugs and her prognosis and she was particularly worried about the possibility of passing the RA on to her two sons. Pain was her worst symptom and she was keen to learn ways to deal with it.

A programme of PE was designed to fit in with her attendance for IM MTX and monitoring. It was agreed that Wendy's primary problem was the pain in her knees. This was addressed first and backed up with a pain information leaflet (Figure 4.3). During the next 10 weeks she underwent the PE programme and she incorporated exercise regimes and pacing and prioritizing into her daily activities. She learned how to cope with a flare and by the end of the programme felt that she could control her pain to an acceptable level.

Within 12 weeks a combination of the efficacy of the MTX and the PE programme had transformed her disease and her attitude to it. By the time she returned to the hospital for her outpatient appointment she felt that she was in control of her disease rather than it being in control of her. Her PE programme was documented and when she saw the CNS she was able to share this alongside her shared-care card. Joyce is still making good progress, has joined her local Arthritis Care group and is currently involved in the ASMP.

What causes pain in rheumatoid arthritis?
Pain is the first thing that people notice when they get rheumatoid arthritis (RA). It can start in just one joint or in a number of joints. One of the causes of this pain is inflammation. When there is little inflammation, you often feel less pain. However, this is not the whole story. Other things such as anxiety, depression and fatigue (tiredness) can make pain feel worse or become harder to control.

Does pain have a purpose?
Yes, it does. It stops us from hurting ourselves. For instance, a child will drop a hot object before he/she is badly burnt. Pain is also the way our body tells us that there is something wrong with it. If we are in a lot of pain, or the pain carries on for some time, we usually go to the doctor who puts a name to the problem. However, the pain from RA is different. It seems to forget what it came for! The pain tends to become 'chronic'. Chronic pain is pain that lasts longer than six months. This kind of pain can be harder to control than short-term pain.

How much pain should I feel?
Pain is a very personal experience. People with the same disease may have different levels and types of pain. This means that someone with a very bad RA may feel less pain than another person with mild RA.

The amount of pain you feel does not only depend on how active your RA is. It can also change when you become interested in what you are doing or what is going on around you. Many people find that their pain is worse when they are sitting alone doing nothing, or are in bed in the dark where there is nothing to take their minds off it. People often feel less pain when they are doing something that they enjoy. Pain can also change from day today. Doing too much can cause this; for example, overdoing the housework or rushing around at work. Very often it seems to change for no reason at all.

Will I get rid of my pain?
Most people with chronic pain never get rid of it altogether but that does not mean that it cannot be kept at a reasonable level. Of course what is 'reasonable' is different for each person. For example, someone with a high pain tolerance may not wish to take pain-killing tablets, even if their pain is severe. Those who do not like taking drugs may prefer to take fewer painkillers but put up with more pain.

At the end of the day the pain belongs to the person who feels it. It is up to you to decide what you can live with. The doctors and health carers are there to advise you about the kinds of pain relief there are. It is up to you to choose what you would like to try.

What kinds of drugs will help?

* analgesics;
* non-steroidal anti-inflammatory drugs (NSAIDs);
* steroids
* anti-depressants.

(contd)

What else will help my pain?

Other things that may help are:

- massage;
- relaxation;
- distraction;
- splinting;
- heat.

Heat

Heat will not cure pain, but many people find it very comforting. There are two types of heat, *dry* and *moist*.

Examples of *dry* heat include:

- *electric pads:* These are used if you have just one or two painful joints;
- *electric blankets:* These are good if you have pain all over;
- *hot water bottles:* Good for just one or two painful joints. Some people prefer to use a hot water bottle rather than a pad as they feel the weight of the bottle on their joints helps;
- *hot/cold packs:* These are easy to use. They can be heated in a microwave oven or in hot water. They mould to the joint and are easy to keep in place with a towel.

Examples of *moist* heat include:

- *hot shower or bath:* Very good at relieving 'all over' pain. Make sure that the bathroom and your towels are warm. This will help to prolong the good effects of the moist heat;
- *wash basin or bowl of hot water:* A good method of helping to reduce pain in the hands or feet.

You can use any of these methods of dry or moist heat to ease the pain but do follow a few simple safety rules.

- *Always* protect the skin with a towel or cloth before applying a hot water bottle.
- *Never* use boiling water.
- *Always* follow the safety guide which comes with electrical appliances.

Cold

Some people find that they get better pain relief by using cold therapy. The most common methods are:

- *bag of frozen peas:* Useful for larger joints such as knees or elbows. They mould well to the joint when kept in place by a towel;
- *hot/cold packs:* Useful for larger joints. Can be kept in the freezer.

To use the above methods, cover the joint with a cloth or towel. This will stop you getting an ice burn. Place the peas or the pack over the joint and then wrap a towel around it to keep it in place. Leave it in place for about 10 to 15 minutes.

- *Never* use ice on your hands or feet if you have poor circulation.

Massage
Massage can be a very potent painkiller. It can be done for you by your partner or a friend, or if the joint is easy to reach, you can do it for yourself. Always use massage oil as you can break or stretch the skin. This can be bought quite cheaply from a chemist or stores such as the Body Shop. Some people prefer to use aromatherapy oils, but these should be used with caution. Some essential oils can have a bad effect if you are taking blood pressure tablets or are pregnant. If you are not sure, ask your doctor, nurse or chemist.

Relaxation
Relaxation really can help you to overcome pain. There are very good scientific reasons for this. Unfortunately, it is not easy to learn how to relax and it is even more difficult to relax when you are in pain! You usually learn from audio-cassettes and many hospitals will either give you one or record one for you. You can only learn these methods by practice and it may take a number of months before you are really good at it.

Distraction
Some people who have chronic pain are able to use this method for a few hours each day. Others can only do it for short periods. The idea is to take your mind off the pain by concentrating deeply on something. This can be hard to do when you are in pain.
    Methods of distraction are:

- *Visual distraction:* Look through a magazine and choose a picture that you like. Look at it closely and then start to describe it out loud in detail. When you have done this, close your eyes and try to describe it again from memory. Let your mind run free and try to think if the picture reminds you of a place or holiday that you have had. Go over this in your mind. As you get better at it, you will find that you can distract your mind away from your pain.
- *Hearing distraction:* Many people find this method of taking their mind off their pain very useful. It works best if you can use a personal cassette player and listen through earphones. Choose a piece of music that you like and try to concentrate on it. When the pain gets worse, increase the volume. If the music makes you think of any images such as waves breaking on a beach, follow them through. If you don't like the music, choose a talking book or a funny tape; humour is a great way to distract your mind from the pain. This is a very good way of helping when you are in bed in the dark.
- *Social distraction:* Good company can divert your mind from your pain so do try to get out as much as possible or invite your friends to visit you. Make it

(contd)

clear that you may have to ask them to leave if it gets too much. This is not a slur on their company, it is just one of the difficulties you have with your RA. You need to help them understand your problems.

Rest

Pain can make you feel more tired than usual. If you are always in pain, or if the pain has woken you in the night then you are going to feel pretty tired! When you feel more tired you will find it more difficult to control the pain. The best way to control your pain is to take more rest. Don't feel guilty, you are not being lazy. You have good cause to feel tired. Try to pace yourself and take periods of rest after each spate of activity. It is a good idea to make yourself lie down on a settee or bed for set periods of time each day. Try adding one of the other pain-relief methods, such as relaxation or distraction. Try to spoil yourself a little – after all, it is all part of the treatment.

Splinting

It is a good idea to rest any joint that is very painful. A good way to rest a single joint is to wear a splint. A splint will stop your making movements that cause pain. It can also prevent the pain from starting. If you are wearing splints all day, you should remove them every two hours and do some gentle range-of-movement exercises. This will help to stop the joint becoming stiff.

Combining different methods

As you can see, there are many different ways of reducing your pain. Most people find that they get the best relief by not just staying with one method. They get better results by using a number of different methods at the same time. A good example is to take non-steroidal anti-inflammatory tablets and analgesics, but also to use relaxation and heat. There are many things you can try so if one combination does not help, try another.

Take control of your pain – don't let it control you

Remember

- Pain is a personal experience, it belongs to the person who feels it.
- No two people have the same pain and it is for you to decide what you can stand.
- Use more than one method of pain control. If it does not work, try another.
- Take your anti-inflammatory drugs regularly.
- Take analgesics before the pain gets too severe. They work better this way.
- If you are in a lot of pain take your analgesics regularly and don't be frightened to take the maximum amount if you do not need to.
- Rest if you feel tired. This will help you to control the pain.
- Do not give up. If one method does not help, always try something else.

Figure 4.3 Patient information: pain in rheumatoid arthritis.
Source: Hill (1998).
Reproduced with kind permission of Churchill Livingstone.

Some Common Questions

Q4.8: At what stage should I start the PE process?

This is a difficult question to answer. Many people suggest that an early, intensive programme can achieve the greatest reduction in disability (DeVellis and Blalock, 1993). This seems to make sense. Learning coping skills at the start of the illness journey should help patients for the rest of their lives. In practice this is not always the right time as many patients undergo a period of grief or bereavement reaction when they learn they have a diagnosis such as RA, and they may be in a state of denial. It has been suggested that trying to educate patients at this stage can be counter-productive and lead to further depression (Donovan et al., 1989). If this occurs, the correct intervention is probably counselling. When the patient starts to ask questions about his/her disease and treatments, PE can commence.

Q4.9: What if the patient wants to discuss another topic rather than what is planned?

The skilful nurse can usually incorporate the patient's wishes. For instance, if you have planned to address exercise and the patient wants to discuss pain, you can meet both aspirations by discussing the effects of exercise on pain levels and include the need for prophylactic analgesia.

Q4.10: How will I know if he/she has taken the information in or learned the taught skill?

The easiest way is by patient feedback. You can do this through starting each session by asking if he/she has any questions from the previous session or how he/she got on with the relevant task over the last week. If the patient had agreed to master a skill such as a stretching exercise, ask him/her to demonstrate it.

Q4.11: If I only have a short session, what should I teach?

You will need to make a list of items and place them in an order of priority. For instance, if a patient with OA needs to lose weight, rather than teaching him/her everything about diet and exercise you might present the patient with a list of weight-reducing strategies such as not eating between meals, grilling rather than frying, not eating after 8 pm, and reducing fat and sugar intake. Ask the patient to choose two or three behaviours he/she believes he/she can accomplish and agree a contract to be adhered to until your next session.

> **Q4.12: If I am teaching a group of patients, should I mix the newly diagnosed patients with those who have had the disease for many years?**

It is better to teach newly diagnosed patients in a separate group but include patients who have had the disease for a long time as lay teachers, because they can act as good role models.

Summary

PE is one of the most important aspects of the nursing care of patients with rheumatic diseases, and it is accepted by all health professionals as an effective component of total patient management. Many of the rheumatic diseases run an unpredictable course, with periods of exacerbation and remission. Patients need to be able to tailor their treatments to their day-to-day disease activity, and the knowledge that PE provides enables them to self-manage their condition safely and effectively. Dargie and Proctor (1998) have shown that nurses working in the primary health sector can make a unique contribution to care in this area, and it is hoped that other nurses working in the field will follow their example.

Chapter 5
How Can Health
Professionals Help?

Patients with rheumatic diseases require complex and multifaceted treatment regimes if their physical, social and psychological needs are to be met successfully. No single profession has the ability to provide for all their needs and so the expertise of a number of health professionals is necessary. Not all health professionals are mentioned in this chapter, as their advice will be the same for a person with arthritis as for someone with any chronic disease and the community nurse will be well versed in their roles. However, each patient is an individual, and even when two patients have the same diagnosis with similar severity their treatment plan may differ. Knowing who provides what, and when it is appropriate to refer, comes with experience. This chapter is written to point those working in primary care in the right direction.

Q5.1: Why does the nurse have the central role?

Of all the professionals involved in the care of patients it is usually the nurse that patients contact when they have a problem. This is the case whether they are attending the hospital, their local surgery or are seen at home. Most patients describe nurses as being easy to talk to and approachable, and many nurses have been in post for a number of years and so patients feel the nurse 'knows them well'. This 'one-to-one' relationship is particularly important when managing patients with chronic conditions, as it lays the foundations of a reciprocal trusting relationship that is necessary for therapeutic nursing care.

Over recent years practice and community nurses have been encouraged to utilize and develop their skills to become more autonomous, innovative practitioners carrying out expanded roles. This encompasses health promotion and ill-health prevention, and includes those features given in Table 5.1.

Table 5.1 Functions of the present-day practice nurse

Provide therapeutic nursing care
Raise health consciousness
Teach
Practice anticipatory care
Act as a patient advocate

Source: Hyde (1995).

Providing they are given adequate education and training nurses can occupy a central position (Figure 5.1) in the care of rheumatic patients, undertaking a large proportion of the management, routine follow up and education of these patients. An excellent example is the innovative nurse-led, community-based arthritis clinic at Sonning Common Health Centre near Reading (Dargie and Proctor, 1998). The aims of the clinic are outlined in Table 5.2.

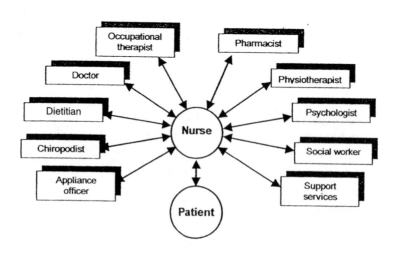

Figure 5.1 The role of the nurse in the multidisciplinary team.

Table 5.2 Aims of the community-based Arthritis Clinic, Sonning Common Health Centre

To provide an easily accessible service for the assessment, support, education and monitoring of arthritis patients and their families

To help patients to participate in preventing the deterioration of their condition, maintain its stability and cope with its effects on their day-to-day lives

To develop a specialist arthritis resource for patients and fellow team members

To strengthen links between the community and the local hospital rheumatology department

To encourage other practices to set up similar initiatives

Q5.2: How should I assess the rheumatic patient?

Making an accurate assessment of the patient's symptoms and problems will enable the nurse to make correct referrals to other members of the multidisciplinary team. The assessment will need to include:

- disease symptoms;
- physical function;
- psychological status;
- knowledge of the disease and its treatments;
- social function.

It is suggested that management record forms similar to the one described in Chapter 7 are used as a template for accurate record keeping.

Disease Symptoms

The most notable symptom of the rheumatic diseases is pain, and this is why the majority of patients make an appointment with their general practitioner (GP) (Symmons and Bankhead, 1994). Other symptoms include:

- joint swelling;
- joint stiffness;
- generalized fatigue.

There are a number of tools available to assess their severity and subsequent relief (Table 5.3). Examples with references of each are provided in Chapter 7.

Table 5.3 Tools for assessing rheumatic symptoms

Ritchie Articular Index	Tenderness and swelling (rheumatoid arthritis only)
Daily diary cards	Pain, stiffness, fatigue
Body maps	Pain, swelling
Skeletal maps	Joints affected
Joint count outline	Pain, swelling

Physical Function

Effect on function can be life altering and it is important to be able to make a quick but accurate assessment. Two widely used question-naires are available:

1. The Stanford Health Assessment Questionnaire (HAQ) – purely physical function ;
2. The Arthritis Impact Measurement Scales (AIMS) – physical function, psychological status, pain.

The HAQ was originally developed in the USA (Fries et al., 1980) but it has been adapted for British use (Kirwan and Reeback, 1986). It has the advantage of being very quick to complete. The AIMS (Meenan et al., 1980) was also developed in the USA and has a British version (Hill et al., 1990). It takes longer to complete than the HAQ but includes more domains. Both are completed by the patient and so could be sent to them prior to their consultation. The HAQ is a 0–3 scale and the AIMS is 1–10, the higher the score the worse the function. Patients who have a high score on either may need to see the physiotherapist, occupational therapist or social worker.

Psychological Status

Chronic, painful diseases can cause psychological distress, some patients becoming anxious and others depressed. Patients with rheumatological disease have a higher incidence of depression than the general population (DeVellis, 1993). The AIMS questionnaire includes individual anxiety and depression scales that can be combined to provide an overall assessment of psychological status. The higher the score, the worse the psychological status.

The Hospital Anxiety and Depression Scale (HAD) was devised by Zigmond and Snaith (1983) for use in the general population in patients who do not have a diagnosed depressive illness. It consists of 14 questions, seven on anxiety and seven on the depression scale. Scores of 8–10 suggest a borderline psychological condition, and 11 or above indicates the necessity for further intervention such as a psychological or psychiatric referral.

Patient Knowledge

Knowing what the patient understands about his/her disease and treatment is fundamental to patient-centred care. Patients have their own value systems and their lay beliefs are part of that system (Donovan et al., 1989). Care must be seen as relevant to them or they will not participate. For instance, when deciding whether to take their drug therapy, patients compare the potential side-effects and efficacy with the severity of their symptoms and act accordingly (Donovan and Blake, 1992). The Patient Knowledge Questionnaire (Hill et al., 1991) is a well-validated tool for rheumatoid arthritis (RA) that is short and quick for the patient to complete. This can be used prior to the start of patient education (PE), and repeated on completion of the programme. An increased score will show accumulation of knowledge.

Social Function

The AIMS questionnaire is helpful here as it contains items about difficulty getting around the community, using transport and communicating with friends and relations. A low score indicates few problems.

One area that requires investigation by verbal questioning is sexual function. This is an important aspect of many people's lives but it is better to ask the patient directly. The practice nurse has an excellent opportunity to broach the subject with female patients who attend for cervical screening. The opportunity is less obvious for male patients but a simple question such as 'some men with arthritis have problems with their lovemaking, have you found this to be the case?' tells the patient that it is a subject you are happy to discuss. An ideal opening exists when discussing the side-effects of sulphasalazine, as this can cause a reduction in the sperm count.

Make sure this important area is not forgotten in both young and older patients. If they do not want to talk about it they will soon let you know. For further information read Prady et al. (1998).

Q5.3: How important is rest for the rheumatic patient?

Fatigue is an ever-present symptom for many patients and they need to know how and when to rest. There are two types of rest applicable to rheumatic patients:

1. whole-body rest;
2. specific joint rest.

Obtaining a sensible balance between physical activity and rest is a real challenge for both patient and health professional. Whole-body rest is particularly important when systemic, inflammatory disease such as RA is present, as active inflammation causes energy depletion. Rest also protects organs and systems from pathological stress experienced during illness. In addition to restorative nightly sleep, patients may need to rest during the day. However, it is point-less telling a patient he/she 'should take plenty of rest'; the prescription of rest should include some definite instruction such as:

* where to rest;
* when to rest;
* how long to rest;
* how often to rest;
* correct positioning.

It is unusual to recommend total bed rest, but diseases such as polymyositis and polymyalgia rheumatica may occasionally require this.

Q5.4: How much rest does the patient need?

At stages of acute inflammatory activity, 8–10 hours of night sleep and an additional 30–60-minute rest during the morning and afternoon. Specific joint rest is discussed in the section on splinting.

Q5.5: How can physiotherapy help?

The most important contribution of the physiotherapist is to assess patients' neuro-musculoskeletal functional ability and plan a programme of treatment. When referring the patient the information should include:

- the diagnosis;
- disease duration;
- disease progression;
- presenting problems.

Treating patients with an arthritic disease is often problematic, as the clinical presentation can be different for each patient and the course of the disease is frequently unpredictable (Smruti Riley, 1998). The patient encounters multiple problems (Table 5.4) and the goals of treatment are to:

- reduce pain;
- reduce stiffness;
- reduce fatigue;
- increase range of motion;
- attain the optimal level of function;
- prevent further deformity.

Q5.6: What treatments do physiotherapists use?

Physiotherapists have an array of treatments at their disposal (Table 5.5) and the one chosen as most appropriate for the condition must also be suitable for the individual patient. Patients with a rheumatic disease may well have had a number of different types of treatment. They know what they have responded well to and also what has been unsuitable, and this must be taken into account during the assessment. It is also important that patients realize that physiotherapy is a form of self-care requiring their commitment and involvement, rather than being something that 'is done to you to help you get better' (Stamp, 1998).

Table 5.4 Problems encountered by patients with arthritis

Limited range of movement
Reduced muscle strength
Decreased endurance
Functional limitations
General debility
Gait abnormalities
Poor posture

Table 5.5 Physiotherapy treatments

Exercise
Thermal treatments
Ultrasound
Acupuncture
Transcutaneous electrical nerve stimulation (TENS)
Hydrotherapy
Traction

Q5.7: How can exercise help?

Exercise is vital if optimal function is to be achieved and it can also help to reduce pain, fatigue and depression (Bunning and Materson, 1991; Strenstrom, 1994). There are several types of exercise including:

- stretching exercises;
- strengthening exercises;
- aerobic exercises.

All have been shown to be safe and to have therapeutic benefit even for those with arthritis of the weight-bearing joints such as the hips or knees. A more detailed explanation is given in Smruti Riley (1998).

Simple Apparatus

There are some cheap and simple aids that can help in the exercise regime. A soft ball or plasticine can be used to increase hand function. Light ankle weights or weight-training equipment can add extra resistance. Pulley systems can be used on either arms or legs.

Q5.8: Is a home exercise regime beneficial?

Many patients, for instance those with RA and osteoarthritis (OA), need to incorporate exercise into their daily routine. Although it is undoubtedly beneficial, exercise can also be painful, boring, tiring and time consuming, making it rather difficult to adhere to on a regular basis. Patients need to be convinced that daily exercise is an investment in their future and most importantly:

- believe that exercise has positive benefits;
- have confidence in their ability to carry out the regime.

It is better to start with a short, easy programme and slowly build it up. Incorporating goals and functions that are important to the patient will aid compliance and give the patient confidence in his/her ability.

Q5.9: What are thermal treatments?

There are two forms of thermal treatment:

1. heat;
2. cold.

Although neither of these therapies will have any effect on the underlying disease, their therapeutic benefit lies in their ability to reduce pain, stiffness, swelling and muscle spasm (Lehmann, 1990). Anecdotal experience suggests that it is preferable to use ice in the acute stages of inflammation and heat during the chronic phase. However, there is no real consistency in the research as to the specific use of heat or cold and so it is probably best to concur with patient preference.

Q5.10: How does heat therapy work?

Heat can be used in either its dry or moist form (Table 5.6). Some therapists advocate the use of wax baths, and these are fine when used in a physiotherapy department. However, attempting to use hot wax at home can be very difficult and hazardous as the hands are usually painful and dysfunctional, and many patients have reported burning themselves.

Table 5.6 The application of heat

Dry heat	Moist heat
Infra-red lamps	Shower
Hot water bottles	Contrast baths
Heated pads	Heated pool
Microwave packs	Moist packs

Patients can apply local heat to any part of their body, and if they have generalized pain immersing themselves in a warm bath or taking a shower will help. Heat should be applied for approximately 20–30 minutes.

Q5.11: How does cold therapy work?

Cold therapy reduces pain, swelling and inflammation. It reduces pain in three ways:

- blocking nerve conduction;
- decreasing muscle spindle activity ;
- releasing endorphins.

Swelling is reduced by vasoconstriction, which decreases blood flow and capillary pressure. Cold lessens inflammation by blocking the release of histamine.

Q5.12: How is cold therapy applied?

Cold is applied via ice packs, cool packs, iced water and vapocoolant sprays. Patients who apply ice at home can apply a bag of frozen peas to a joint as this is cheap and moulds well to its shape. Crushed ice can be placed into a polythene bag wrapped in a damp towel. The ice can be left in place for between 10 and 30 minutes.

Q5.13: What are the contraindications for cold therapy?

- Patients should be warned never to place ice directly onto the skin as this can cause an ice burn; they should always apply a flannel or tea towel first.
- Patients with impaired circulation should not use ice therapy.
- Raynaud's phenomenon is aggravated by cold and so this form of therapy should not be used.
- Hypersensitive patients can exhibit urticaria.

Q5.14: What is ultrasound?

Ultrasound is a form of sound wave that penetrates deep into the structures and the sound oscillation produces a local, concentrated heat within the tissue. This exerts an analgesic effect and also increases blood flow to the area (hyperaemia), which enhances the collagen fibre separation. The result is increased extensibility of the connective tissue, allowing greater stretch (Lentall et al., 1992). The use of ultrasound is contraindicated in acute inflammatory conditions, but once patients reach the sub-acute phase it can help to improve their range of movement when given in conjunction with stretching exercises.

Q5.15: Does acupuncture have a role in treatment?

Acupuncture originated in China, where it has been used for hundreds of years. Specially designed needles are inserted into acupuncture points on the body. They can be stimulated manually by lifting and turning the needle or mechanically by attaching the needles to a machine that vibrates them (Cawthorn and Billingham, 1998). The mode of action is thought to be the enhancement of the production of endorphins, which reduces pain. Acupuncture is advocated by some physiotherapists and some GPs, particularly for patients with OA (Bird, 1993).

Q5.16: What is transcutaneous electrical nerve stimulation (TENS)?

TENS is a non-invasive therapy in which electrical current is applied via electrodes placed on the skin. The most commonly used types of TENS unit are:

- high frequency (15–150 Hz);
- low frequency (2 Hz).

High frequency is thought to work by stimulating A fibre activity. The theory is that this closes the 'gate' (Gate Control Theory) and so inhibits the transmission of painful sensations via the C fibres to the brain. This higher frequency is thought to bring swifter pain relief than low-frequency TENS.

Low-frequency TENS works by stimulating the production of endogenous opiates and is thought to have a more long-lasting effect than high-frequency TENS.

The value of TENS for the relief of pain has been demonstrated in a number of different types of arthritis including OA (Aubin and Marks, 1995), RA (Kumar and Redford, 1982) and ankylosing spondylitis (Nienhuis and Hoekstra, 1984).

TENS can be used in both acute and chronic conditions, is self-administered, safe and easy to apply. The only real side-effect is an allergic reaction to the electrode gel or tape.

Q5.17: How useful is hydrotherapy?

The role of hydrotherapy is to help to mobilize and rehabilitate the patient. It works at different levels by:

- raising the body temperature;
- reducing joint stiffness;
- inducing muscle relaxation;
- reducing joint load.

The buoyancy of the water allows the patient to move more freely and increase his/her range of motion, and the warmth of the water induces analgesia. Hydrotherapy also has the advantage of allowing the patient to exercise multiple joints simultaneously.

The disadvantage of hydrotherapy is that it is not widely available and some patients improvise by attending their local swimming baths.

Contraindications for hydrotherapy include:

- unstable cardiac impairment;
- severe respiratory conditions;
- open wounds;
- agoraphobia;
- some skin conditions.

Q5.18: When is traction used?

This form of treatment is sometimes used for back and cervical spine problems. It can relieve pain and is undertaken on both inpatients and outpatients.

Q5.19: How do walking aids differ for different rheumatic diseases?

Walking aids can relieve the patient's pain by decreasing pressure on the affected joints. They can also give physical support, which provides much needed confidence in their ability to mobilize. The physiotherapist usually provides walking aids, and the choice of the most suitable appliance can be a complicated business. For instance, patients with OA of the lower limbs will probably need a conventional round-handled stick but someone with RA whose hands are affected will require a stick with a special moulded handle, as in a Fisher stick (Figure 5.2).

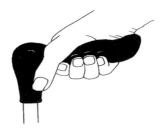

Figure 5.2 Fisher stick.
Reproduced with kind permission of Geoff Hill.

Some patients will not be able to use either and alternatives are:

- zimmer frames;
- pulpit frames;
- gutter crutches.

Many patients buy their own walking stick. Unfortunately they often choose one of the wrong height and frequently hold it in the wrong hand.

To measure the correct length of a walking stick, place the stick upside down with the handle resting on the floor. The bottom end of the stick should reach the patient's wrist when they are standing upright wearing their outdoor shoes. When holding the stick for use, the elbow should be flexed at 30° when the patient is standing normally.

A walking stick should always be held in the hand on the opposite side of the body to the affected joint.

It is very important to check that the rubber feet of walking sticks are not bald, thus having no grip on the ground.

Q5.20: What help can occupational therapists offer?

Occupational therapists are trained to appraise both the physical and psychological consequences of disease. They are multiskilled and able to assess and plan many different types of intervention (Table 5.7). They often visit the patient in his/her home or working environment to make their assessment.

Table 5.7 Occupational therapy skills

Activities of daily living assessment
Home adaptation assessment
Teaching joint protection techniques
Teaching energy conservation techniques
Stress management techniques
Provision of orthotics
Provision of assistive devices
Workplace assessment

Q5.21: What does joint protection involve?

When joints and their surrounding structures are inflamed they become more vulnerable, and if the joint involved also happens to be one of the smaller joints such as the fingers, they are even more so. The objectives of joint protection have been described by Hammond (1994) as the:

- relief of pain;
- reduction of both internal and external joint stress;
- reduction of inflammation.

There are eight basic principles underlying joint protection (Table 5.8), and providing they are adhered to there are few activities that someone with a rheumatic disease should not carry out. It is not the type of activity a person undertakes that can be detrimental; it is the way in which they perform it that matters.

Table 5.8 Principles of joint protection

Always use the largest joint possible
Distribute the strain over as many joints as possible
Do not force joints into deforming positions
Use orthotics to protect, support and rest the joint
Use gadgets and labour-saving devices
Do not hold joints in the same position for any length of time
Avoid gripping objects tightly
Listen to your body

It is important to note that it is difficult to change the way in which everyday activities are carried out. However, it is worth the effort as there is evidence that patients who attended a joint protection course did use assistive devices, and this resulted in a reduction in their pain (Nordenskiold, 1994). Examples of such devices are shown in Figure 5.3.

Q5.22: What are orthotics?

Orthotics is the correct name for splints. Splints can be supplied by the occupational therapist, physiotherapist or appliance fitter and are of two types:

- working splints;
- resting splints.

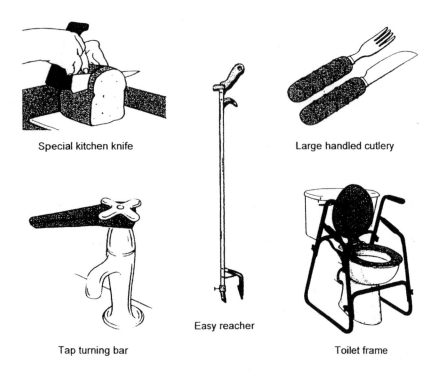

Special kitchen knife

Large handled cutlery

Tap turning bar

Easy reacher

Toilet frame

Figure 5.3 Assistive devices.

Working splints

As the name implies, a working splint allows a patient to use a joint without placing it under undue stress. A futura wrist splint is a good example of a ready-made working splint (Figure 5.4). This is worn when undertaking everyday activities such as vacuuming, ironing or driving a car. It is composed of an elasticated splint with a metal insert to the palmar aspect of the hand/wrist. The insert is moulded to the individual hand, holding it in the optimal supportive position. It is held in place by velcro fastenings.

This type of splint should not be worn continuously as it can lead to muscle weakening. If the patient needs to wear it for any length of time, it should be removed two-hourly and the joint should be put through a gentle full range of motion exercise before it is replaced. For patients who need to place their hands in water, splints made entirely from plastic are available.

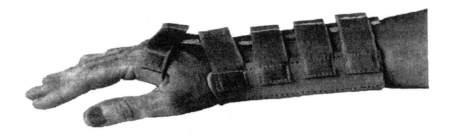

Figure 5.4 Working wrist splint.

Resting splints

These are usually worn on the hands or legs at night by patients with inflammatory arthritis. They keep the limb in a good position whilst at rest and so delay the onset of joint deformity. However, if the joint is in a flare they can be used during the day to rest it. They are made to measure for each individual from a thermoplastic material moulded to the joint. Resting splints differ from working splints in that they encase the whole of joint and do not leave the digits free (Figure 5.5).

Resting splints are needed for both the right and left side and it is impractical to wear them simultaneously, as this makes activities

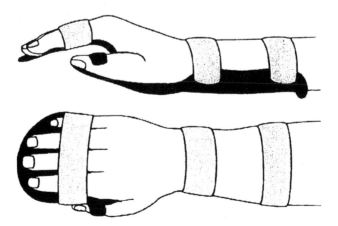

Figure 5.5 Resting splint.

such as going to the bathroom impossible. Patients should be advised to wear just one of the splints on alternate nights.

Another type of resting splint is a soft cervical collar that is sometimes supplied to patients who have pain in the cervical spine. A soft collar is not suitable for daytime use, as it does not provide adequate support. Cervical collars should not be worn constantly unless they are used to support atlanto-axial subluxation.

Q5.23: What advice should be offered to the patient for conserving energy?

Fatigue can be one of the most debilitating symptoms of rheumatic disease and is often associated with disease activity. As a general rule, the more inflammation present, the greater the fatigue. However, inflammation is not the only cause of fatigue and other causes include:

- chronic, unremitting pain such as that experienced by some patients with OA;
- anaemia due to poor diet or chronic blood loss associated with non-steroidal anti-inflammatory drugs;
- disturbed or poor sleep patterns.

Whatever the cause, patients need to conserve the energy they have to accomplish the activities that are most important to them; therefore, undue expenditure needs to be eliminated. In general there are four basic ways in which energy can be conserved (Table 5.9).

Table 5.9 Energy-conservation techniques

Pacing oneself
Prioritizing activities
Efficiency measures
Correct posture

Q5.24: What does pacing mean?

One of the most frustrating aspects of rheumatic diseases is their unpredictability; patients may feel very well one day and very ill the next. This makes advanced planning of daily activities extremely difficult and their inclination is to do as much as possible on the day that they feel well. Unfortunately they usually pay for it the following day. Patients need to assess how they feel each morning and then write themselves a daily activity list, spreading tasks evenly and interspersing them with frequent periods of rest. It is important that patients are taught not to overestimate their abilities, as setting themselves unachievable goals will only lead to further frustration.

Q5.25: What advice should patients be given about pacing?

Prioritizing activities

The patient is the only person who can decide what the most important elements are in his/her life. It is unlikely that he/she will be able to undertake everything he/she wishes to on a given day. When listing their activities, patients need to place them in order of importance so that if they do not meet all their goals, those they consider the most important have been undertaken.

Efficiency measures

Energy is a finite resource and expending unnecessary energy needs to be eliminated. For instance, if the patient can plan the day so he/she only has to go up and down stairs once or twice, this will save energy. Using electrical equipment when possible and carrying out activities such as preparing food or ironing in a sitting rather than standing position will help.

Correct posture

Poor posture can waste energy and inefficient lifting and handling techniques need to be assessed. Kitchen surfaces and cupboards should be at the correct height to avoid undue bending and stretching, and getting in and out of chairs and beds should not cause undue exertion.

Q 5.26: What is the role of the appliance fitter?

The appliance fitter can supply some commercially made orthotics such as futura splints and some cervical collars. They usually dispense callipers for patients with unstable ankles, and knee braces for those with unstable joints that are unsuitable for a surgical procedure. Patients who suffer osteoporotic crush fractures are occasionally prescribed corsets to use until bone-bulking agents and analgesics become effective.

Patients with rheumatic diseases often have foot problems. For instance, those with RA develop deformities of the metatarsophalangeal joints, or the foot spreads and they can suffer from fallen arches. The appliance fitters can measure the foot and provide extra deep or wide surgical shoes with specially designed insoles. Not all shoes need to be made to measure. Patients with OA of the lower limbs can be provided with trainers and insoles to reduce impact loading (Figure 5.6). The nurse can refer direct to an appliance fitter.

Q5.27: How important is podiatry?

Foot problems are common in the rheumatic diseases and can lead to:

- pain;
- lack of mobilization;
- ulceration;
- changes to gait;
- poor posture.

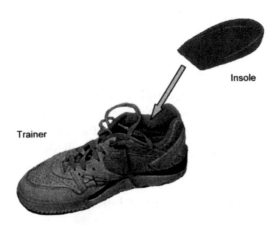

Insole

Trainer

Figure 5.6 Impact-absorbing footwear for OA.

Podiatrists are highly skilled and many undertake postgraduate training to become surgical podiatrists, who are able to carry out procedures such as straightening hammer toes and correcting hallux valgus. The goals of the podiatrist in relation to the rheumatic patient have been articulated by Widdows (1998), and are shown in Table 5.10. Referring a patient to the podiatrist or chiropodist can lead to a greatly improved lifestyle.

Table 5.10 Goals of treatment by the podiatrist

Reduction of callosities and corns
Redistribution of body weight from metatarsal heads by use of orthoses and insoles
Protection of bony prominences
Prevention of lesser toe deformities
Reduction of shock to the legs and feet
Promotion of a normal gait
Reduction of the risk of ulceration
Advice on footwear

For example, patients with RA often develop callosities under the MTPs that cause pain on walking. The simple procedure of paring them down will greatly reduce the pain and aid mobilization. Another common problem is the erosion of the metatarsal heads, which many patients describe as 'walking on pebbles'. The addition of a rubber metatarsal bar fitted to the underside of the shoe may reduce the stress and lessen the need for surgical removal of the heads.

Rheumatoid nodules can appear almost anywhere on the foot, but the most common sites are:

- plantar surface of the heels;
- beneath the metatarsals;
- top surface of the toes;
- Achilles tendon.

The constant pressure can lead to ulceration and as the foot is usually in an ideal environment for bacteria to proliferate, the ulcers can become infected. The podiatrist will be able to reduce the risk if patients are referred at an early stage.

Q5.28: Can diet help in the treatment of rheumatic disease?

People with rheumatic diseases face particular dietary problems as, in addition to their disease symptoms, physical disabilities may make it difficult for them to shop and prepare their meals (Ryan, 1995c). A well-balanced diet is essential, as a well-nourished body will recover more quickly from the ravages of frequent flares and ill health that rheumatic patients often endure. For a more in-depth discussion read Douglas and Byrne (1998).

Q5.29: Is a special diet advised for patients with RA?

RA has been linked with food intolerance and a number of studies have shown similar results (Darlington et al., 1986; Van der Laar and Van der Korst, 1991), which have been collated by Pattison (1998) and include:

- Food sensitivity is found in about 30% of patients.
- Food sensitivity appears to be associated almost exclusively with RA.
- Food-fasting diets relieve symptoms after three or four days.
- Reintroduction of food causes a flare in the symptoms.

If patients think a particular food flares their RA it is best to advise them to exclude it from their diet for about a week and then reintroduce it. If the symptoms subside and reappear when the food is reintroduced this could be a coincidence, so they need to repeat the exercise three times before they can be sure they are intolerant to the food. Obviously foods that cause a problem should be avoided.

Q5.30: What is the benefit of essential fatty acids (EFAs)?

Evidence is emerging that oils containing EFAs reduce the formation of pro-inflammatory prostaglandins and so reduce the symptoms of RA. There are two main groups of EFAs:

- omega-3   found in fish oils;
- omega-6   found in plant seed oils.

Eicosapentanoic acid (EPA) and docosahexanoic (DHA) are the two main omega-3 EFAs and fish oil capsules containing high concentrations can be bought at chemists' and health food shops. However, they are expensive and a better idea is to incorporate pilchards, mackerel, sardines or salmon into the diet three or four times a week.

Gamma-linolenic acid (GLA) is the most common omega-6 EFA and the most usual source is evening primrose oil (EPO) but current research shows that it is efficacious only at large doses, such as 8–10 capsules a day (Cleland and James, 1997).

EPO is available on prescription for psoriasis, but is not prescribed for RA. The quality of EPO is variable and should come from a reputable source, but is expensive for patients to buy.

Q5.31: Will a particular diet help patients with OA?

There is no specific diet that helps the symptoms of OA, but obese patients will profit from weight reduction (see Q2.6 and Q2.18). Recent research suggests that losing about 5 kg reduces a person's risk of developing OA of the knee over the subsequent 10 years by 50% (McAlindon and Felson, 1997). Weight maintenance can also be problematic as patients in pain and with reduced mobility have difficulty exercising. Patients with OA should be referred to a dietitian or provided with dietary advice that is both realistic and achievable.

Q5.32: How will diet affect prognosis in osteoporosis?

The production and retention of normal healthy bones relies on a well-balanced diet that is rich in calcium and vitamin D.

Calcium

The richest source of calcium can be found in dairy products and skimmed milk. A diet with sufficient calcium should include:

- low fat yoghurt;
- cheese;
- broccoli;

- spinach;
- tinned salmon;
- tinned sardines.

In addition a pint of skimmed milk should be consumed each day. Without these foods, a normal diet usually provides about 500 mg of calcium each day, which is less than that recommended (Table 2.11). Some special diets such as high fibre and low calorie regimes are also low in calcium and may require supplementation.

The rate of calcium absorption is decreased during illness and with ageing and it is important that the calcium intake takes account of this. The approximate calcium content of some common foods is shown in Table 5.11.

Table 5.11 Calcium content of common foods

Food	Calcium content (mg)
Pint whole milk	660
Pint semi-skimmed milk	690
Small carton low-fat yoghurt	285
4 oz cottage cheese	80
2 oz hard cheese	380
4 oz tinned sardines	620
8 oz baked beans	120
Two slices white or brown bread	66
Two slices wholemeal bread	36

Some patients are unable to tolerate dairy products and their diet can be supplemented with soya milk fortified with calcium. Those who are unable to obtain an adequate calcium intake from food should consider calcium tablets. Vitamin D is usually given with calcium as it facilitates its absorption.

Vitamin D

The most natural source of vitamin D is of course sunlight, but unfortunately sunlight can be in short supply in the UK! The skin also loses its ability to convert ultraviolet light into vitamin D after the age of 50 and supplementation may be necessary from cod liver oil and halibut oil capsules. Dietary vitamin D can be obtained from:

- liver;
- cheese;
- oily fish.

It is also added to cereals, low-fat spreads and margarine.

Q5.33: Should certain foods be avoided in gout?

Although drug therapy has largely replaced special diets in the treatment of gout, it is sensible to restrict the intake of foods high in purines, which are shown in Table 5.12.

Table 5.12 Foods high in purines

Animal-based foods	Fish	Vegetables
Liver	Anchovies	Peas
Kidneys	Crab	Spinach
Heart	Herrings	Lentils
Sweetbreads	Mackerel	Whole-grain cereals
Meat extracts	Roe	
(Oxo and Bovril)	Sardines	
Yeast extracts	Shrimps	
Paté	Whitebait	

Protein such as meat should be eaten in moderation and alcohol should be restricted. Weight control is important and losing a few pounds if overweight will help to control the gout by decreasing urate levels. However, the timing of starting a reducing diet is crucial as periods of food restriction following an attack of gout may provoke another. Crash diets for extremely obese patients are also inappropriate as this causes ketosis, which raises urate concentration and exacerbates an acute attack.

Some Common Questions

Q5.34: Should I advise patients to rest or exercise?

It depends on their condition. For instance, if a patient is in a flare of their RA, it is better to rest the joint and just carry out passive range-of-movement exercises to prevent joint stiffness. Once the flare has passed, more active exercise should be encouraged.

Q5.35: Can patients with arthritis of the hips and knees do activities such as walking, running, dancing and climbing stairs?

Yes, stationary bicycling, walking and low-impact aerobic dancing is safe even when the joint is symptomatic.

Q5.36: Should patients carry heavy loads up and down stairs?

The patient should not attempt to carry loads greater than 10% of their body weight as this significantly increases loading at the hip.

Q5.37: Are TENS units safe to use in pregnancy?

The use of TENS during pregnancy is not advocated.

Q5.38: Should I refer patients with gout to the podiatrist?

It depends. Following an acute attack of gout, the skin around the joint often peels off and if the area rubs on shoes it can become infected. The podiatrist can help by offering advice about relief of pressure and well-fitting shoes.

Q5.39: Are there any biochemical tests for food allergy?

There are no reliable tests for food allergy at present. Enzyme-linked immunosorbent assay (ELISA) has a scientific basis as it looks for immunoglobulins in the blood; however, it is not very accurate at present. Cytotoxic testing also involves a blood test and is unreliable.

Q5.40: Are there any side-effects from EFAs?

Taken in large doses they can cause nausea and vitamin A toxicity.

Q5.41: Patients often ask about green-lipped mussels and selenium ACE; are they efficacious?

There is no evidence to support their use in arthritis.

Summary

The rheumatic diseases are complex and often difficult to manage and so require the knowledge and skills of the multidisciplinary team to obtain the patient's optimum outcome. Community nurses can play a central role in coordinating the team and making appropriate and timely referrals. To do this, they need a clear understanding of the diseases and knowledge of the elements of care provided by other health professionals. Knowing when, what and how to utilize the skills of other team members is an essential part of the art of nursing the rheumatic patient.

Chapter 6
Psychosocial Aspects of Rheumatic Diseases

Rheumatological conditions can have a multifaceted effect on all domains of function. There are the obvious physical elements of pain, stiffness and fatigue, but the consequences of illness are far reaching, impacting on the social and work arenas as well. Illness often has its greatest impact on those areas we value most. For example, a person who has been a regular football player and is no longer able to engage in this activity will experience feelings of loss relating to this activity and find it difficult to cope with the void left by no longer being able to play football. It is therefore essential that nurses do not concentrate solely on the physical manifestations of the condition but also address psychological and social needs that will ultimately affect well-being. Living with a condition such as rheumatoid arthritis (RA) has been described as 'the tightrope between freedom and a life sentence' (Maycock, 1988).

Chronic Illness

Q6.1: What are the features of chronic illness?

Chronic illness has been defined as an altered health state that will not be cured by a single surgical procedure or a short course of medical therapy (Miller, 1992). Reif (1975) identifies three main features of chronic illness:

1. The disease symptoms interfere with normal activities and routines, e.g. a patient with arthritis can experience losses in social

146

relationships, a disruption of leisure activities and limitations in the workplace (Yelin et al., 1987).

2. The medical treatment can be limited in its effectiveness. There is no cure for RA. The aim of treatment is to reduce symptoms such as pain and stiffness and suppress the disease process. Disease-modifying anti-rheumatic drugs (DMARDs) take many months before efficacy can be assessed and even when the condition is under control the patient may still experience the daily symptoms of the condition. Also, a patient may experience a toxic reaction to the drug therapy that would necessitate its discontinuation even if it were proving effective in dampening down the condition. This can exert a heavy psychological toll on the patient who re-experiences the symptoms of illness. Patients have to cope continually with a state of uncertainty about the symptoms they will experience and the outcome of treatment interventions.

3. Treatment, although intended to mitigate the symptoms and long-term effects of the disease, contributes substantially to the disruption of the usual pattern of living. Many patients will require ongoing blood tests to monitor the safety and efficacy of their drug treatment; this can create problems if a patient's occupation allows no flexibility for time off.

Q6.2: What reaction will a patient have to being informed that he/she has a chronic rheumatological condition?

Patients with RA (and other rheumatological conditions) will require time to adjust to their alterations in everyday functions. It is not uncommon for patients to remain in a state of denial about the condition for anything up to five years (Le Gallez, 1993).

Krueger (1984) relates disability to loss and states that the patient will go through several stages, which include:

• shock;
• retreat, denial or disbelief;
• grief, mourning or depression;
• hostility and anger;
• adjustment.

Case Study

Ann is a 34-year-old woman with two young children. She works part time in a shop. She has been told that she has RA. She remembers feeling bewildered when the consultant told her the diagnosis as she had always associated arthritis with older people. Ann is determined to carry on as normal and not make any allowances for the condition. She feels she is far too busy with the family and her job to have time to be ill.

Ann is distressed to find that she always seems to be in pain and feels constantly tired, she is no longer able to keep up with the housework and seems to be more short tempered with the children. The consultant has arranged for Ann to see the nurse specialist.

In this situation the nurse specialist can spend time learning more about Ann and her day-to-day life so that her needs can be placed in context. The nurse can begin to explain to Ann the symptoms that she may be experiencing at the moment. These can include:

- *generalized pain;*
- *stiffness, predominantly in the morning;*
- *fatigue;*
- *loss of appetite;*
- *low mood;*
- *weight loss.*

It is important that the nurse enables Ann to identify the problems that particularly relate to her individual circumstances, so that care management can be implemented that has meaning and relevance to Ann. This may include advice on pain management, pacing activities, reducing fatigue and acknowledgement of altered emotional state.

This initial meeting will be the first of many and Ann will probably require regular guidance, support and advice from the nurse whilst the condition is in an active phase. Further encounters will include explanations regarding the objective of drug therapy and evaluation of the care that has been initiated such as pacing of activities. The nurse's role is not to pressure Ann into the realization of her condition but to provide educational care and support that matches Ann's identified needs.

As the nurse–patient relationship develops, the sharing of information will help to minimize natural fears and anxieties. Any advice offered will pass through a filter of lay beliefs, which are rational to the person who holds them and can change following new experiences and exposure to information. It is important to encourage Ann (when she feels able) to participate in as many treatment decisions as possible. When an individual chooses a course of action (e.g. pacing activities; cleaning a different room in the house every day instead of cleaning the whole house in one day) he/she is more likely to own it and stick with it even if the beneficial effects are not immediately apparent. Informing patients (and their significant others) about treatment options and enabling them to choose from the alternatives will heighten their sense of control and may in fact play a key role in whether or not the treatment actually has a beneficial effect (Wallston, 1993).

If Ann's condition requires DMARD therapy to suppress the disease process, a choice of potential agents should be offered so that Ann is actually involved in the decision-making process.

Q6.3: What is the effect on self-esteem when you have a condition such as RA?

Self-esteem is the basis from which humans in our culture function, with emphasis placed on youthfulness and fitness. Physical difficulties and disabilities experienced can be potentially stigmatizing and adversely affect self-worth (Maycock, 1988).

Pigg et al. (1985) define self-esteem as how one feels about oneself: 'It is a concept that assigns a value to who one is, how one wishes to be and how one thinks others see and expect one to be'. A person with an inflammatory condition such as RA has a potential for physical changes and altered function to occur. Therefore perceived body image, regardless of whether it is associated with a visible change, is likely to be a problem. When the signs of the condition are intrusive the person has to work at creating a resemblance of normal life and this can be perceived as further evidence that the person is different. The likely causes of a negative internal perception include:

(a) the changes brought about by the disease itself such as a physical change in appearance, e.g. ulnar deviation of the finger joints. Shaul (1995) carried out in-depth interviews in 30 women with

RA and found that a noticeable concern about deformity existed. The women in the study were fearful that the swelling they observed would not subside and that their joints would permanently assume an unnatural shape;

(b) the visibility of the treatment programme. Medications which can alter physical appearance include prednisolone and neoral;

(c) the patient's perception of how others see his or her body as being different. The patient will require access to a practitioner with counselling skills who can encourage the patient to acknowledge concerns he/she may have regarding his/her body image. This may include the involvement of a psychologist or clinical nurse specialist in rheumatology with advanced skills. Concerns about body image must be addressed and managed in such a way as to minimize the effects on day-to-day functioning.

Q6.4: What is the effect on mood in patients with chronic inflammatory rheumatological conditions?

The exact prevalence of major depression in RA is not known but it is estimated to range from 21% to 34% (Creed et al., 1990). The exact incidence may in fact be a lot higher than this as it can often be undiagnosed in patients with RA, especially as some of the symptoms of active inflammatory arthritis overlap with the signs of depression such as loss of energy. We therefore need to employ a method for assessing depression so that it can be identified and treated appropriately.

The role of the nurse must be to identify depressive symptoms in these patients and refer to the appropriate source (Table 6.1 lists the symptoms associated with depression). Some nurses are equipped with the necessary skills and knowledge to help patients through a depressive episode, especially if the depression is related to an increase in disease activity. Some patients will require the additional intervention of antidepressants and may benefit from referral to a psychiatrist or psychologist.

Major depression has been defined by Parker and Wright (1995) as that which is a profound, depressive syndrome of sufficient intensity to impair psychological, social and vocational functioning. Moldofsky and Chester (1970) describe two types of depression:

- a depression which was more marked when joint tenderness was at its peak;
- a depression which was more marked when joint tenderness was better. This latter type of depression has a less favourable outcome.

Table 6.1 Symptoms associated with depression

A loss of interest and enjoyment in life
A lack of drive and motivation
Fatigue
Agitation and restlessness
Alteration in appetite
Alteration in sleep pattern
Loss of self-confidence
Feeling worse at a particular time of day, usually mornings
Irritability
Feeling useless, inadequate

Depression can accompany pain, sleep disturbance and fatigue in patients with RA (Nicassio and Wallston, 1992; Shaul, 1995). One participant in Shaul's research stated, 'It's a vicious cycle with RA, you feel depressed so your arthritis acts up more and the more it acts up the more depressed you get until it breaks you somehow'. Patients who were unable to maintain gainful employment also reported higher levels of depression (Newman, 1993).

Case Study

Danny is a 40-year-old man with RA. He has recently lost his job and feels he is no longer useful to the family as he can no longer provide financially for their needs. He has worked since leaving school and now finds he is alone all day with nothing to do. He describes feeling 'horrible' on waking and it is an effort to get up every day. Danny feels useless and disorientated. He is referred to the nurse specialist for advice and support. At the first meeting he is withdrawn and mentions that he is coping in his own way and doesn't want to talk about it. The nurse spends time talking to Danny about his family, hobbies and past experiences so that she can begin to know Danny as a person.

After the hour session, Danny asks if he can come next week. The nurse arranges this and over the next month Danny gradually describes how the loss of his job has made him feel; he doesn't have many social contacts outside the family and he has felt isolated, alienated and frightened. Time is spent concentrating on the things in life that Danny can do, and self-esteem begins to return. An appointment is made with the disablement resettlement adviser and Danny is offered a place on a training course, which he is keen to accept.

Although Danny required a lot of support after the initial trauma of loss of employment he now only contacts the nurse if his symptoms flare up or he finds himself in a situation where he is unable to cope. He has also become an active member of the local Arthritis Care group and has become involved in arranging social events for other people with arthritis.

Q6.5: What is the effect of depression on life activities?

Depression is associated with a reduction in valued activities (Yelin and Callahan, 1995). Women with RA surveyed by Reisine et al. (1987) reported limitations in their ability to perform general household cleaning activities or go shopping. Katz and Yelin (1995) found that persons with RA who had depressive symptoms performed 12% or fewer of valued activities compared with people with RA who were not depressed.

Q6.6: What is the relationship between depression and isolation?

Isolation, often associated with depression, is a destructive mechanism. Prior to the onset of illness the patient has an understanding of his/her role both in social interaction and in work. This societal role may now be lost, changed or at least no longer clear (Pigg et al., 1985). Speed of decline or setback can be associated with social withdrawal, and people living with disability report a greater sense of isolation and alteration than those in non-disabled control groups (Harper, 1983).

The Family

Q6.7: How will the family be affected?

The family has a crucial role to play in health (see Table 6.2) and an equally pivotal role to fulfil when one of its members experiences illness.

Table 6.2 Functions of the family unit

Sexual well-being
Emotional support, e.g. love and affection
Physical assistance with everyday tasks
Recreational activity and social commitments

Affleck et al. (1988) state that the family will be affected in one of three ways:

(1) The arthritis brings the family unit closer together. The support offered from within the family will influence the individual's coping ability and play a major part in compliance with treatment and rehabilitation. The importance of the family role in patient outcome was illustrated in a study focusing on the impact of behavioural intervention to minimize pain in patients with RA. The intervention incorporating family support was more effective in reducing pain than the intervention with the patient alone (Radojenic et al., 1992).
(2) The family experiences minimal alteration in role responsibility.
(3) There is a negative effect on relationships between family members as a consequence of illness. The change of role is recognized by the majority of female patients but by only a minority of male patients. Men largely accept the role of caring for their female partner. However, whilst the female partner is as willing as the male to accept the responsibility of caring, some male patients are unable to accept this offer, viewing it as a threat to their perceived role as head of the house and family provider (Le Gallez, 1993).

The family plays a central role in the success of treatment and management, and its members require education about the condition and treatment interventions to adopt an active role in decision making. If family members are not aware of the importance of pacing activities, a patient's resting time may be conceived as lazy and wasteful, leading to unnecessary friction within the family unit at a time when there will be great uncertainty and disruption.

Prior to the onset of illness family members will have adopted different roles within the unit, which may need renegotiating. This can be a time of great uncertainty for all concerned, with feelings of helplessness occurring throughout the family structure. The nurse will need to act as a mediator, facilitating discussions about role alteration with appropriate family members. This is of vital importance as spouses of patients with RA can have a poor perception of the disability, pain and stiffness their partners live with (Phelan et al., 1994).

Q6.8: What activities within the family will be affected?

Activities within the family can be divided into two main areas:

- instrumental activities which include cooking, cleaning, financial management and shopping;
- nurturing activities including making family arrangements, maintaining family ties, looking after members and listening to others. It is this area of activity that has highest value to the individual and the family (Reisine, 1995).

Conditions such as RA and osteoarthritis (OA) can impact on both of these aspects of family activity, with patients reporting the most difficulty in areas of shopping, cleaning and maintaining family ties (Yelin et al., 1987). It is at this level of individual participation that arthritis often has its greatest impact as far as the patient is concerned.

Often the depth of impact depends not only on the degree of disability but also on how well each patient is able to adjust to the disease and accept the physical limitation it imposes (Le Gallez, 1993).

Q6.9: Is communication within the family unit affected?

The impact of any chronic illness on the family unit can lead to a breakdown in communication. Research has shown that children living with a parent who had RA were afraid of developing the disease but had not communicated this fear to their parents (Le Gallez, 1993). Misunderstandings and silences such as these reinforce the need for education. Maycock (1988) refers to a young patient with newly diagnosed RA who complained that due to her arthritis not being visible her family could not comprehend the severity of the illness. It is not unusual to experience conflict within the family, especially feelings of over-protectiveness on the one hand and anger and resentment at the disruption of existing family life on the other. Some patients may find it easier to discuss their situation more openly with friends, who can be viewed as offering support without having to take full responsibility for the consequences.

Q6.10: What is the effect on marriage?

Many studies have demonstrated that married people have fewer health problems and a lower mortality rate than individuals who are single, divorced, separated or widowed (Reisine, 1993). In a study of patients with RA the women who were married experienced greater feelings of being needed, physical affection and assistance with practical tasks than those who were not married (Manne and Zautra, 1989). Obviously marriage alone will not guarantee support. It is the quality of the marital relationship that is important and not surprisingly high levels of spouse criticism are directly related to maladaptive coping behaviour.

Q6.11: How are sexual relationships affected?

Patients with RA report a loss of sexual interest and reduced sexual satisfaction (Blake et al., 1987). Patients often attribute difficulties in their sexual relations directly to the arthritis and its treatment (Ryan, 1996). Factors found to have a negative effect on sexual activity include pain, fatigue, limitations in joint movement, medication and reduced opportunities for sex (Le Gallez, 1993; Ryan, 1996).

The nurse has been cited by patients as the person whom the patient is most likely to approach to discuss any sexual problems. Therefore the nurse must receive adequate training, support and ongoing supervision to be an effective practitioner in this area. The reasons why nurses do not often assess the impact of illness on sexuality are given in Table 6.3.

There are several organizations that can provide both verbal and written support in this area. These include Arthritis Care and the Association to Aid the Sexual and Personal Relationships of People with Disability (SPOD). The addresses of these organizations are included in Chapter 7. It has to be the nurse's responsibility, despite the apparent difficulties in assessment, to ensure that patients have access to these services.

Table 6.3 Problems associated with the assessment of sexuality

Taboo subject – embarrassment for both the patient and nurse
Lack of training, education and supervision for nurses
Lack of time
Lack of privacy in the clinical environment

Q6.12: What is the effect in the family on children with a parent who has arthritis?

Hirsch and Reich's study in 1985 found that the self-esteem of adolescent children living with a parent who had arthritis was lower than that of children living with healthy parents but no different than that of those children whose parents also have long-term conditions such as depression.

For adolescents living in a family with a disability there is greater opportunity for friends to view the family in a negative light. However, Le Gallez (1993) found that 75% of children living with a parent with RA experienced a minimal impact on their lives, and in some cases it had the positive effect of bringing the family closer together with the children expressing deep concern and displaying a nurturing attitude towards the ill patient. The 25% of children who felt living with a parent with arthritis was detrimental could be divided into two groups:

- those whose parents were unable to accept the pain and physical limitations;
- those children who resented the fact that a parent was ill and as a result showed little consideration and compassion for them.

Q6.13: What benefits does social support offer to patients with RA?

The right level of social support has a major impact on an individual's ability to cope with the condition. The function of social support is shown in Table 6.4.

The advantages of such support include:

- increased self-esteem (Fitzpatrick et al., 1988);
- decreased depression (Revenson and Majerovitz, 1991);
- increased performance of positive health behaviour;
- increased self-management activities.

Table 6.4 The functions of social support

Expressing positive affect
Encouraging communication of feelings
Providing information and advice
Validating beliefs, emotions and actions
Enhancing psychological well-being
Providing material aid

Q6.14: Can social support have any negative effects on patients with RA?

It is very important that the support offered matches the support needs perceived by the patient. If there is a disequilibrium between support needs and support offered then the following may occur:

- Patients may resent the degree of support offered, reinforcing the concept of powerlessness.
- The family may become over-protective by encouraging the patient to rest continually rather than engaging in specific exercises. This will have the negative consequences of increasing pain, stiffness and muscle wasting.
- The patient can become over-dependent on the family, adopting disability as a way of life and ceasing to be an active participant in care management.
- The patient may be less likely to seek help if he/she feels unable to return the support. This can cause a reduction in the patient's self-esteem.
- Support can become a form of social control (Rook, 1990).

Q6.15: How helpful can support groups be?

Support groups can provide an additional source of support as well as providing the environment to learn more about self-management techniques. For some patients support groups remove the potential for isolation and provide a regular point of contact with people who may be experiencing similar difficulties. Those attending the group and who are coping well can serve to act as role models and motivators for these individuals coping less well. Details of support groups around the country can be obtained from Arthritis Care and the Arthritis Research Campaign.

Work

Q6.16: What effect do rheumatological conditions have on an individual's ability to work?

The experience of chronic illness will not only affect biological functioning but also impact on societal roles. RA is responsible for a reduction in work status, and individual and family income. After the condition occurs, 59% of patients with RA lose their employment and those that remain in employment earn only about 50% of the income expected for them based on their age and educational level (Yelin and Callahan, 1995).

Q6.17: What is the impact of not working?

- The individual faces the loss of income as well as the effect on psychological functioning.
- Family members may find their own employment is affected by the circumstances. This may necessitate either leaving the workforce to provide care, or entering the workforce to compensate for lost income.
- Society incurs a financial burden, as it must meet the cost of unemployment. In the UK, patients with a back disorder account for one-seventh of all sickness invalidity benefit payments (Frymoyer and Cats-Baril, 1991). It is the relationship between the limitations caused by the condition and the requirements of the job that will influence whether a particular individual is able to carry on in his/her present occupation. If an individual is employed in manual work but finds him/herself in a situation where it is difficult to lift objects because of the pain he/she is experiencing in his/her upper limbs, he/she may face the fact that he/she is no longer able to continue in his/her present job.

When an individual finds him/herself in this situation it is important that he/she is given time to adjust to this proposed radical change in lifestyle. This is especially so in conditions such as RA that most commonly occur in the third or fourth decade of life as patients may face many years without being able to work. The degree of interference that RA has on a person's ability to work is equivalent to that found in patients with multiple sclerosis (Devins et al., 1993).

- The patient may require counselling to cope with the loss experienced by not being able to work and may require referral to other agencies, including the disability employment adviser for information on retraining and the social worker for advice on benefits.

People with a musculoskeletal disorder are more likely to stop working if they are:

- older;
- female;
- have fewer years in education;
- have pain and co-morbidity;
- have experienced limitation in function (Yelin and Callahan, 1995).

Control Strategies

Q6.18: How can the nurse help the patient to achieve a sense of mastery over the condition?

To achieve a sense of mastery the patient must obtain a degree of empowerment over the situation and develop control strategies to cope with the changing nature and symptoms of many of the rheumatological conditions. Langer (1983) defines control as the active belief that one has a choice amongst responses that are differently effective in achieving the desired outcome.

Q6.19: What are the different models of control theory?

1 Locus of control

This model originates from Rotter's (1966) social learning theory, which states that behaviour is related to outcome. If a patient believes that a particular behaviour will achieve the desired outcome he/she will continue to engage in it. For example, if a patient finds that by participating in a regular exercise programme joint stiffness is reduced, then the individual is more likely to carry out this behaviour than an individual who perceives no benefit from exercise. The locus of control concept separates individuals into two groups. Those who believe that control over outcome is dependent on their own behaviour are referred to as having an internal locus of control. Those individuals who believe that control over outcome is dependent on the action of other people or simply a matter of luck or chance are referred to as having an external locus of control. This latter group has been shown to be associated with less favourable clinical outcomes (Bishop et al., 1990) and often portray a lack of self-involvement, denial of the situation and an avoidance of information.

Patients newly diagnosed with RA may need to rely on the support, education and guidance of others but as they become more familiar and have more experience of the condition it may be appropriate to begin the development of coping strategies to adopt an internal locus of control. RA is characterized by flares and remission and a patient may experience a fluctuating locus of control. If a flare of the condition is experienced the patient may need to rely on the support of family members until the symptoms have subsided, enabling the individual to reinstigate self-management techniques.

2 Learned helplessness

This concept is related to psychological adjustment in patients with chronic RA (Callahan et al., 1988). If a patient has not been able to influence outcomes with previous behavioural interventions such as relaxation therapy which has not reduced pain levels, further attempts to reduce symptoms may be regarded as futile and a belief develops that the reduction of symptoms is not within one's individual control. Higher levels of helplessness as recorded on the rheumatology attitude index (RAI) relate to low self-esteem, lower levels of formal education, impaired functional ability and increased anxiety and depression.

3 Self-efficacy

Self-efficacy is based on beliefs about control and refers to personal judgements, not actual performance of behavioural outcome. For example, I might believe I could climb Everest even though I have never attempted this. It is important that a patient believes that he/she can implement a given behaviour to achieve a certain outcome otherwise he/she will not attempt it. If a patient does not believe that exercise will influence the pain and has reservations about being able to perform the exercise programme, the programme will not be undertaken.

Perceived self-efficacy can reduce depression and pain as well as enabling the individual to obtain a degree of control over his/her condition (Lorig et al., 1989). Self-efficacy is situation specific and therefore learning techniques can be employed to achieve the outcome. In the area of pain management, members of the study group given cognitive and relaxation instructions were better able to control the pain than the control group.

4 Cognitive control

An individual who understands what is involved in a process or event may not be able to prevent it occurring but may be able to cope with it owing to an increased understanding. If a patient does not know what to expect when a flare of RA occurs, he/she may well become distressed and feel helpless because of the increase in pain and fatigue. If a patient knows to expect these symptoms, although still unpleasant, the anxiety will be reduced and the patient may feel more able to cope with the situation.

Q6.20: What do patients require to feel in control of their condition?

In coping with arthritis patients are helped by three factors (Affleck et al., 1988). These are:

- being given the opportunity to express feelings and concerns;
- receiving encouragement, hope and optimism;
- receiving advice and information.

The nurse therefore needs to provide the following type of support:

- emotional – sharing feelings and concerns;

- instrumental – arranging for care interventions;
- information – providing advice.

Arthritis and Pregnancy

Q6.21: Is arthritis a contraindication to pregnancy?

Arthritis itself is not a contraindication to pregnancy and has no added foetal complications. The decision whether to start a family is likely to be influenced by:

- personal preference;
- disease activity;
- social support;
- finances.

Potential parents often express concern about the likelihood of offspring inheriting the condition. Although it has been shown that there is a slight increase in the frequency of RA in first-degree relatives with the condition, there is no means of predicting whether a child will develop the condition (Le Gallez, 1995).

Q6.22: How is antenatal care best managed?

Once pregnancy has been established, time must be spent deciding the best management plan for the woman and the baby. Most drug therapy is contraindicated during pregnancy (see Q3.16 and Q3.39), and the nurse will advocate other methods to minimize joint symptoms.

During the antenatal phase the nurse will need to provide support and information to the expectant mother and family, which will include:

- *pacing activities*: Fatigue is normal in pregnancy but may be compounded by disease activity so there needs to be a balance between rest and activity. Fatigue can be heightened in the first trimester and following delivery. Good quality sleep, gentle exercises and early maternity leave are all important (Richardson, 1992);

- *coping with pain:* Relaxation can be helpful, together with the application of hot and cold therapies. The occupational therapist can provide advice on joint protection and the suitability of proposed baby equipment.

In RA 75% of women experience some remission in their symptoms during pregnancy but following birth encounter a return of their symptoms (Le Gallez, 1998). It is therefore important that the mother is reviewed by the rheumatology team soon after the birth to consider the reinstatement of drug therapy to minimize the occurrence of a flare. Patients with ankylosing spondylitis may experience no alteration or an actual increase in their symptoms during pregnancy (Le Gallez, 1995). The consequences of pregnancy are less predictable in patients with systemic lupus erythematosus. If the condition is in an active phase then close monitoring of renal function will be required.

Q6.23: Are there any problems with labour?

A normal vaginal delivery can be expected except where the woman has hip involvement which restricts hip abduction (Richardson, 1992). It may be necessary to support the joints with pillows throughout the labour to minimize discomfort. If a Caesarean section is indicated, the mother with RA will require a cervical collar to prevent hyperextension of the neck.

Q6.24: What advice should be given postnatally?

The support of the community rheumatology sister and the health visitor will be essential in providing physical and psychological support. Education may be required on:

- *lifting the baby:* A cot height is required that minimizes bending. Wrist splints may reduce pain when handling the baby;
- *dressing the baby:* Clothes with Velcro will be easier to fasten;
- *establishing a routine* that accommodates both the mother's and the baby's needs.

Conclusion

This section of psychosocial aspects has highlighted the important role of the nurse. If such issues are not identified and addressed they will have negative consequences on well-being. The nurse must be proactive in this area in order to provide a patient-focused service that has both meaning and relevance for patients and their families.

Chapter 7
Assessments, Guidelines and Further Information

This chapter contains information that may be useful to the community nurse but is not included in other parts of the book. It focuses on:

- guidelines;
- recording sheets;
- patient assessments;
- useful addresses.

Guidelines

A number of sets of useful guidelines have been produced. The British League Against Rheumatism (BLAR, 1997) has produced the first ever nationally agreed standards of care for arthritis in both the primary and secondary sector. There are two distinct types of standards:

- essential;
- desirable.

The Royal College of Nursing (RCN) has produced guidelines on administration of intramuscular (IM) gold, IM methotrexate (MTX) and administering intra-articular (IA) injections.

Q7.1: What are the essential standards applicable to primary care?

1. A general practitioner (GP) should both discuss the nature of the arthritis and examine the joints at an early stage in patients with osteoarthritis (OA) or rheumatoid arthritis (RA).

2. A GP should explain the role of the following:
   - exercise: OA and RA;
   - weight control: OA and RA;
   - footwear/chiropody: OA only;
   - analgesia: OA and RA;
   - non-steroidal anti-inflammatory drugs (NSAIDs):   OA and RA;
   - disease-modifying anti-rheumatic drugs (DMARDS):   RA only;
   - oral steroids/injectable steroids: RA only;
   - physiotherapy: RA only;
   - the hospital (rheumatology or orthopaedic department) in treatment/care of arthritis: RA only.
3. The local pharmacist should be able to offer clients the choice of non-child-resistant caps on their medication containers for patients with both OA and RA.
4. Physical access to the following environments should be ensured for patients with OA and RA:
   - GP surgeries;
   - local/community pharmacist ;
   - people's homes;
   - all public buildings;
   - all public transport vehicles.

Q7.2: What are desirable standards for primary care?

1. A GP should explain the role of:
   - the hospital (rheumatology or orthopaedic department) in the treatment/care of arthritis: OA only;
   - physiotherapy as a possible treatment   OA only;
   - steroid injections as a possible treatment   OA only;
   - social workers   OA and RA;
   - someone able to discuss personal and/or sexual relationships   OA and RA;
   - footwear/chiropody as a possible treatment   RA only;
   - the rheumatology nurse practitioner   RA only.
2. A GP should provide written information for patients with RA and OA on:
   - arthritis in general;

- medication being taken for arthritis;
- exercise;
- voluntary self-help/support group;
- self-management courses.
3. Additional information/advice should be made available to patients with RA or OA about:
   - arthritis and the workplace;
   - placing, assessment and counselling team (PACT) and the access to work scheme;
   - Arthritis Care and Young Arthritis Care;
   - Arthritis Research Campaign;
   - disabled living centres;
   - social or leisure activities.

Further information about the standards is provided in the BLAR report entitled *Standards of Care – towards meeting people's needs*. This report forms part of the larger report *Arthritis: getting it right – a guide for planners*. These documents are available for purchase separately.

Q7.3: What are the RCN guidelines for rheumatology?

The RCN Rheumatology Nursing Forum has produced a number of sets of guidelines to ensure safe and consistent nursing practice.

IM Gold Guidelines

Practice nurses are often asked to monitor the bloods of people with RA who are on potentially toxic drug therapy. The drug most commonly involved is IM gold and the guidelines are shown below.

RCN Guidelines for Administering Sodium Aurothiomalate

1. What is sodium aurothiomalate?

Sodium aurothiomalate (IM gold) belongs to the group of drugs known as slow-acting anti-rheumatic drugs (SAARDs). These drugs suppress clinical and laboratory markers of disease activity and are thought to slow the progression of the disease but the precise mode of action is unknown. Unlike NSAIDs, which produce an immediate therapeutic effect, SAARDs are unlikely to produce any benefit before 12 weeks and often take as long as 24 weeks before improvement is attained.

2. Indications for using sodium aurothiomalate

Sodium aurothiomalate is used in cases of active RA.

3. Contraindications

Females who are pregnant or are breast feeding should not be given IM gold. Likewise those who have gross renal or hepatic disease, history of blood dyscrasias, exfoliative dermatitis or systemic lupus erythematosus.

4. Administration and dosage of sodium aurothiomalate

The drug is given by deep IM injection, followed by gentle massage of the area. An initial test dose of 5–10 mg is usually given and if there are no adverse reactions (skin rash or hypersensitivity), a weekly injection of 20–50 mg given until a response occurs. Most patients will feel no benefit until they have received a total (cumulative) dose of between 500 and 800 mg. Once in remission and providing they do not experience any side-effects, patients are usually maintained on a dose of 50 mg administered monthly, but the physician may vary the dose according to the activity of the disease. If no major improvement has occurred after reaching a cumulative dose of 1000 mg (excluding the test dose) the treatment is usually discontinued although weekly injections of 100 mg for five weeks are sometimes given.

5. Adverse reactions

Side-effects occur in approximately 30% of patients and can appear at any time during the course of the treatment, even after the patient has been successfully treated with sodium aurothiomalate for many years. They are mostly mild, but up to 5% experience severe reactions, which are potentially fatal.

- *Skin:* Skin reactions are perhaps the most common of the side-effects to IM gold and are usually mild. However, if they do develop, the injection should be withheld and their presence should always be reported to the physician, as they may be the forerunners to severe gold toxicity. This side-effect occurs most commonly after a total cumulative dose of 300–400 mg. Rashes may be localized or general and range from minor reactions to major skin lesions. They can mimic almost any skin eruption. Pruritus or 'itching' is quite common and is often first felt between the fingers.

- *Mucous membranes:* Stomatitis and mouth ulcers can develop in some patients. Pharyngitis should raise the question of leucopenia. Patients sometimes complain of a metallic taste in the mouth, which although unpleasant is not a permanent side-effect.

- *Blood:* Thrombocytopenia, neutropenia, agranulocytosis and fatal marrow suppression can develop but the latter is rare. Bruising, particularly around the shins, can be the first indication of thrombocytopenia. A fever and sore throat can indicate the presence of agranulocytosis. Eosinophilia may be an indication of developing toxicity but does not always necessitate stopping gold. The drug manufacturer recommends that a full blood and platelet count are taken before each injection is given and this advice should be meticulously adhered to and the results recorded sequentially. A sudden fall in platelet or white cell count outside normal limits may be reason for the physician to suspend treatment. A fall on three consecutive occasions, even if within normal limits, should also be reported as he/she may wish to suspend or modify the treatment. Blood dyscrasias are most likely to happen when between 400 mg and 1000 mg of IM gold has been given but can occur at any time during treatment.

- *Kidney:* Proteinuria develops in about 10% of patients but is severe in less than 2%. A gradual increase in protein concentration is more significant than a single result and so if protein is detected, do not give the gold but ask the patient to return a few days later for a retest. If the protein persists, consult the physician; it may be necessary to estimate the amount of protein excreted in 24 hours by a more accurate measure than use of dipstix. If blood and protein are present, eliminate the possibility of a urinary infection by collecting a mid-stream urine specimen. If this is negative, the physician may decide to stop the gold.

Rarer side-effects

Rarer side-effects include peripheral neuritis, alopecia and colitis. A small number of patients may experience flushing, nausea or vertigo after an injection.

The nurse's responsibility when giving sodium aurothiomalate

Before beginning the gold injections, you should ensure the patient understands what the treatment is for, how it is to be given, how it will help and what side-effects may occur. It is also important to make sure that the patient knows where the treatment and monitoring will take place, and who he/she should contact if he/she is unable to attend or if he/she experiences any problems. It is always helpful to provide written information to the patient as a back-up to this verbal explanation.

Before each injection:

1. Inspect the skin for rashes and ask if any pruritis has been experienced.
2. Inspect the skin for bruising.
3. Ask the patient if he/she has experienced any soreness of the throat, developed mouth ulcers or loss of taste.
4. Inquire if the patient has experienced any undue bleeding such as epistaxis or bleeding gums.
5. Ask the patient if he/she is experiencing any flu-like symptoms.
6. Ascertain that blood has been taken for a full blood count.
7. Check that the prescribing doctor has seen and approved the results of the previous blood tests.
8. Record the dose given, haematology and urinalysis results, the presence of any unwanted effects and any action taken on the patient's gold card. If the monitoring reveals any adverse effects, withhold the gold and report the symptoms to the doctor.

Q7.4: What are the RCN guidelines for administration of IM MTX?

Drug therapy for patients with RA has changed drastically in the 1990s and the trend is now to introduce DMARDs at a much earlier stage in the disease process. One of the first drugs of choice is MTX; unfortunately some patients have difficulty in tolerating the oral preparation and MTX is prescribed as it has fewer adverse effects. As MTX is given weekly it often falls to the practice nurse to administer and as this is a cytotoxic drug special precautions should be taken.

RCN Guidelines for Nurses on the Use of and Administration of IM MTX in RA

1. What is MTX?

MTX is an anti-metabolite cytotoxic agent. It can be administered via the oral, subcutaneous and IM routes. It suppresses clinical and laboratory markers of disease activity and is used to slow the progression of the disease but the precise mode of action is unknown. Unlike NSAIDs, which produce an immediate therapeutic effect, MTX is unlikely to produce any benefit before 4–6 weeks and often takes as long as 2–4 months before improvement is evident.

2. Indications for using IM MTX

MTX is used in cases of:

- active RA;
- psoriatic arthropathy;
- polymyositis;
- inability to tolerate oral MTX.

3. Contraindications

Relative contraindications:

- abnormal liver function;
- alcohol (increases the risk of liver damage);
- smoking (increases the risk of pneumonitis).

Absolute contraindications:

- pregnancy and breast feeding;
- chronic viral hepatitis.

4. Administration and dosage of IM MTX

Deep IM MTX is given weekly in doses between 5 mg and 25 mg according to disease severity and individual response.

5. Adverse reactions

Side-effects may occur any time during the course of treatment.

- *Gastrointestinal:* Patients may still experience nausea even when the IM route is used. Anti-emetics and/or drug reduction may be considered.

- *Skin:*
  - stomatitis and mouth ulcers can develop in some patients;
  - some patients may experience hair loss;
  - *Herpes zoster* and systemic fungal infections can occur;
  - patients may notice accelerated nodules whilst taking this drug.

Most rheumatologists routinely prescribe folic acid on a daily or weekly basis to minimize the risk of the above side-effects.

- *Respiratory:* Acute pneumonitis is rare but can be life threatening and should be considered if the patient has a dry cough or has experienced recent breathlessness. A sputum specimen must be collected and sent for culture in the event of a productive cough. Incidences of opportunistic infections, such as *Pneumocystis carinii* pneumonia have occurred in patients taking MTX.
- *Blood:* Thrombocytopenia, neutropenia, agranulocytosis and fatal marrow suppression can develop but the latter is rare. Regular monitoring of the blood is required.

- *Liver:* MTX can cause abnormal liver function and hepatic fibrosis. The liver enzyme aspartate transferase (AST), when persistently elevated, is the best guide to toxicity because alkaline phosphatase and gamma glutamyl transpeptidase (GT) may be elevated in acute RA as a consequence of the disease.

6. Drug interactions

Trimethoprim and phenytoin must be avoided because they increase the risk of bone marrow suppression. Be aware that aspirin, acidic NSAIDs and probenecid may increase the risk of toxicity.

7. The nurse's responsibility when giving MTX

Before administering IM MTX each nurse must be aware of the local policy regarding the handling, administration and disposal of cytotoxic agents. Prior to commencing MTX the nurse must check and document:

- that the patient has had a chest X-ray within the last six months (lung function tests may be requested by some rheumatologists);
- that females have received contraceptive advice to avoid pregnancy whilst on, and for six months after taking, MTX;
- fertility – males should be advised that reduced spermatogenesis may occur but is reversible;
- alcohol – patients should be advised to avoid all alcohol because of liver problems;
- smoking – advice should be given to reduce or stop.

Before beginning the injections the nurse should discuss the treatment with the patient, to ensure that he/she understands what MTX is for, how it is to be given, how it will help and potential side-effects. It is also important to make sure that patients know where the treatment and monitoring will take place and who they should contact if they are unable to attend or if they experience any problems. It is always helpful to provide written information to patients to support the verbal explanation.

Before the injection:

1. Ask the patient if he/she has experienced breathlessness, a dry productive cough, mouth ulcers, nausea or any overt signs of infection. The injection should be withheld if any of these has occurred.
2. Ascertain that blood has been taken for full blood count, erythrocyte sedimentation rate or plasma viscosity and liver function tests. A blood test should not be taken until three days after the administration of each injection of MTX as it can take this time for a reduction of the white blood cell and platelet counts to occur. Danger signs include a progressive fall in the haemoglobin, white cells, neutrophils or platelets and abnormal liver function.
3. Check that the prescribing doctor has seen and approved the results of the previous blood test. Some units may have nurse-led protocols that allow the nurse to take the responsibility for carrying this out.
4. Record in the patient's monitoring booklet the dose given, blood results and the presence of any unwanted effects and any action taken. If the monitoring reveals any adverse effects, withhold the MTX and report the symptoms to the doctor. These guidelines should be read in conjunction with the national guidelines for the monitoring of second-line drugs, produced by the British Society for Rheumatology.

Administration and disposal of MTX

- *Administration:* Aseptic technique is essential at all stages. Contact between the nurse and the MTX should be avoided by the use of:
  - thick latex or PVC gloves;
  - plastic apron and water-repellent armlets;
  - safety goggles/mask.
- *Disposal:* Potentially hazardous equipment includes:
  - sharps such as vial, ampoules and needles which should be discarded in the appropriate sharps container according to local policy.

All other disposable equipment including protective clothing should be treated as dry clinical waste and placed in the designated bag according to local policy.

Q7.5: Can nurses give IM injections?

Some nurses have been trained to undertake this expanded activity. The RCN Rheumatology Forum has produced guidelines to ensure that this procedure is undertaken safely.

Guidelines for Nurses on the Use and Administration of IM Injections

1. What is an expanded role?

Role expansion refers to nurses carrying out tasks not included in their normal training for registration. Most of these tasks relate to medical technical interventions usually carried out by doctors.

2. Accountability

The scope of professional practice (UKCC, 1992a) acknowledges that nurses are involved in negotiating the boundaries of practice and should be responsive to the needs of patients and clients. The onus is on each individual nurse to recognize his/her own level of competence and decline any duties or responsibilities unless he/she is able to perform them in a safe and skilled manner. Each nurse is also accountable for maintaining and improving his/her knowledge and should be familiar with the contents of the following documents:

*   UKCC *Exercising Accountability* (1989);
*   UKCC *Scope of Professional Practice* (1992a);
*   UKCC *Code of Professional Practice* (1992b);
*   UKCC *Standards for the Administration of Medicine* (1992c).

3. What are IA injections?

These are injections into the synovial joints. Long-acting steroids are generally used for joint injections and hydrocortisone is used for soft tissue injections.

4. Indications for joint injections

- relief of pain from localized inflammation of the joint for example in RA;
- relief of pain from soft tissue discomfort;
- to aid mobilization;
- to assist with rehabilitation such as physiotherapy;
- to improve function.

5. Contraindications of joint injections

- local infection;
- IA fracture;
- anticoagulant therapy;
- bleeding disorders.

6. Preparation the nurse must undertake prior to the administration of IA injections

The nurse must be able to demonstrate evidence of competence in the administration of IA injections in accordance with the *Scope of Professional Practice* (UKCC, 1992a).

(a) Evidence of competence should indicate that the nurse has knowledge of:
- anatomy and physiology of the joints and soft tissues;
- drugs used and their effects and side-effects;
- indications and contraindications for IA injections;
- potential complications;
- aspiration and injection technique.

(b) Evidence of assessment of competence should be available.

(c) The employer must have precise knowledge of the employee's activities, and agree to them being undertaken by the employee, thereby accepting vicarious liability.

7. The nurse's responsibility when giving IA injections

- obtain written instructions from the prescribing doctor detailing the drug, dosage and site of administration;
- ensure the patient has given informed consent;

- use an aseptic or no-touch technique;
- aspirate the joint if swollen;
- send a sample of synovial fluid for culture if it is very opaque, green or foul smelling;
- if no obvious signs of infection or contraindications are present, administer the prescribed drug into the site stated;
- document the drug, dosage and site of administration in the care records;
- provide the patient with after-care advice.

8. After-care advice

The nurse must advise patients that:

(a) the joint may be painful for 24 hours after the injection. Analgesia should be taken if necessary.
(b) it may take several days before benefit is felt;
(c) the injected joint should be rested as much as possible for 24–48 hours after the injection;
(d) short-term facial flushing may be experienced;
(e) localized skin atrophy may occasionally occur;
(f) the rheumatology department should be contacted if the patient has any concerns.

9. Potential complications following the administration of an IA injection

These are:

- infections;
- damage to the articular cartilage;
- tendon rupture;
- skin atrophy.

Recording Sheets

Q7.6: How should I document my interventions?

Meticulous documentation is essential but it must be quick to complete and yet be comprehensive. The Arthritis Management

Record developed and used at Sonning Common Health Centre by
the practice and district nurse has both of these attributes and this is
shown in Figure 7.1.

SONNING COMMON HEALTH CENTRE ARTHRITIS MANAGEMENT RECORD	Patient label

Date:

Type of arthritis:	Date of diagnosis:

Occupation:	Lives alone yes no Dependents yes no If yes, relationship to patient:

Current medication:

Has had the following X-rays:	Dates	Report

Height (cms):	Ideal weight:

Past arthritic medical history:

Comments from questionnaire:

Pain score:	Depression score:
Sleep pattern:	

ACTIVITIES OF DAILY LIVING ASSESSMENT		
ACTIVITY	COMMENTS	AIDS/DEVICES IN USE
1. Dressing/grooming		
2. Rising		
3. Eating		
4. Walking		
5. Hygiene		
6. Reach		
7. Grip		
8. Activities		

Figure 7.1 Arthritis management record.
Source: Hill (1998).
Reproduced with kind permission of L. Dargie, J. Proctor and W. Bird, Sonning
Common Health Centre.

Education checklist	LFT given	Discussion/date
Disease process		
Drug therapy		
Investigations		
Exercise		
Pain control		
Pain diary Managing a flare		
Joint protection		
Rest, positioning, splinting		
Diet		
Feet and footwear		
Roles of multi-disciplinary team		
Aids/appliances		
Financial benefits		
Coping strategies		
Co-op card needed		
? Depression		
Alternative medicine		

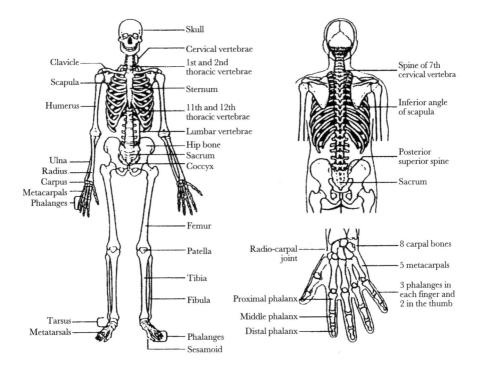

Figure 7.1 (contd)

JOINT PAIN FUNCTION LEVELS

Date	Weight Kgs	BP	PPS	DMS	Daily analgesic	Hb	RAHA	ESR	CRP	Joint pain 1–5 A	B	C	D	Comments/medication

DMS: Duration of morning stiffness   Daily analgesics

PPS: Present pain score (Max = 35)   Total number needed in last week

Joint pain: 1 = No pain
5 = Severe pain

Figure 7.1 (contd)

Patient Assessments

Almost all chronic diseases require some form of assessment for improvement or deterioration, and in general practice it usually falls to the practice nurse to undertake this procedure. Rheumatic diseases are painful, potentially disfiguring and life altering and assessments need to encompass all areas of a patient's life and so should include:

- disease symptoms;
- functional ability;
- psychological status.

Any assessment used needs to be quick and easy to undertake and able to demonstrate trends of change.

Q7.7: How do you measure pain?

This is the most common symptom of rheumatic disease. There are several ways of documenting it and these are discussed in more detail by several authors (Hill, 1998c; Sturdy, 1998b). Useful tools include a simple Daily Diary Card (Figure 7.2), which is completed by the patient for a few consecutive days prior to their consultation.

It should have space to record any activity that exacerbates pain and any therapy or activity that relieves it. The diary card is particularly useful because it can also be used to assess joint stiffness. A body map as shown in Figure 7.3 can be used to indicate the area affected by pain, and if a pain scale is added the intensity can also be measured.

Joint Counts

Diseases such as RA usually involve a number of tender joints and in general the more active joints that are involved, the worse the disease. The Ritchie Articular Index (Ritchie et al., 1968) is used to assess tenderness in RA, and an extra column can also be added to the record sheet to document joint swelling (Figure 7.4).

Pain Diary

Please fill the diary in each day. Record the worst pain that you feel by circling one of the numbers.

1 = no pain
2 = mild pain
3 = moderate pain
4 = severe pain
5 = very severe pain

Please write down any activity that causes or increases your pain, and anything that relieves it.

Please write down the number of painkillers that you take every day.

DATE	PAIN Circle one of these numbers	WHAT CAUSES YOUR PAIN? WHAT RELIEVES YOUR PAIN?	NUMBER OF PAIN KILLERS
	1 2 3 4 5		
	1 2 3 4 5		
	1 2 3 4 5		
	1 2 3 4 5		
	1 2 3 4 5		
	1 2 3 4 5		
	1 2 3 4 5		
	1 2 3 4 5		
	1 2 3 4 5		
	1 2 3 4 5		

Figure 7.2 Pain diary.

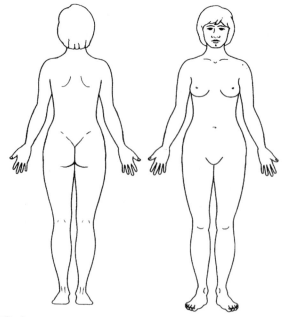

Figure 7.3 Body map.

JOINT		TENDERNESS		SWELLING	
		Left	Right	Left	Right
Temporomandibular Cervical spine					
Sternoclavicular Acromioclavicular					
Shoulder	Left Right				
Elbow	Left Right				
Wrist	Left Right				
MCPs	Left Right				
PIPs	Left Right				
Hip	Left Right				
Knee	Left Right				
Ankle	Left Right				
Talocalcaneal	Left Right				
Midtarsal	Left Right				
MTPs	Left Right				
Total Score					

Figure 7.4 Ritchie Articular Index.
MCP – Metacarpophalangeal joints; MTP – metatarsophalangeal joints;
PIP – proximal interphalangeal joints

Tenderness is elicited by the application of firm pressure to the joints and the response is scored:

- No pain or tenderness reported   0;
- The patient says he/she can feel tenderness   1;
- The patient feels pain and winces   2;
- The patient feels pain and withdraws the joint   3.

The maximum score is 78 but a score of 30 or above is considered to be high. Another method of recording the number of joints involved is the use of a skeletal map (Figure 7.5).

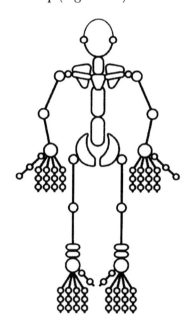

Figure 7.5 Skeletal map.

Q7.8: How do you measure function?

The most frequently used functional index is the Stanford Health Assessment Questionnaire (HAQ) which was developed by Fries et al. in 1980. The HAQ is very quick and easy for the patient to complete and if recorded on a yearly basis will show whether a patient with arthritis is deteriorating or improving functionally. The British version and its scoring system have been validated by Kirwan and Reeback (1986) and a sample of questions is shown in Figure 7.6.

HEALTH ASSESSMENT QUESTIONNAIRE

Name.. Date............................

We are interested in learning how your illness affects your ability to function in daily life. Please feel free to add any comments at the end of this form.

PLEASE TICK ONE RESPONSE WHICH BEST DESCRIBES YOUR USUAL ABILITIES OVER THE PAST WEEK:

	Without ANY difficulty	With some difficulty	With much difficulty	Unable to do
DRESSING AND GROOMING Are you able to: – dress yourself, including tying shoelaces and doing buttons?	☐	☐	☐	☐
– shampoo your hair?	☐	☐	☐	☐

Figure 7.6 Sample of questions which may be included on a health assessment questionnaire.

The Arthritis Impact Measurement Scales (AIMS) were developed in the USA (Meenan et al., 1980). They are a multidimensional tool, incorporating three dimensions that can be used individually or together:

- physical function;
- psychological status;
- pain.

The AIMS takes a little longer than the HAQ to complete and score but has the advantage of being a more comprehensive tool. It has been altered and validated for British use (Hill et al., 1990) and a sample of one of the questions is shown in Figure 7.7. It can be used for almost any rheumatic disease.

Please circle one number
During the past month, about how often did you get together with friends or relatives?

Every day	1
Several days a week	2
About once a week	3
Two or three times in the past month	4
Once in the past month	5
Not at all in the past month	6

Figure 7.7 A sample question from the AIMS questionnaire.

Q7.9: How do you measure psychological status?

Patients with rheumatic disease can become anxious and depressed. This can be assessed by use of the appropriate scale from the AIMS questionnaire or with a tool developed by Zigmond and Snaith (1983) called the Hospital Anxiety and Depression Scale (HAD). The HAD was designed for use in general populations and comprises 14 items on two subscales, seven concerning anxiety and seven depression. High scores on either scale indicate problems. A score of 7 or less indicates no problem, 8–10 is doubtful but 11+ needs to be investigated further. Sample questions are shown in Figure 7.8.

Overall Summary

Rheumatic diseases are numerous, and with an ageing population the numbers affected are increasing rapidly. Their chronicity and life-altering symptoms place an immense physical and psychological

Anxiety

I feel tense and wound up:

Most of the time	3
A lot of the time	2
Time to time, occasionally	1
Not at all	0

Depression

I look forward with enjoyment to things:

As much as I ever did	0
Rather less than I used to	1
Definitely less than I used to	2
Hardly at all	3

Figure 7.8 Sample questions from the HAD.

burden on patients and their families; they also exert a financial burden on the individual and on society as a whole. As a large proportion of these patients receive the majority of their care from the primary sector, the major onus falls on the primary health care team. Nurses have a central role in caring for such patients. For instance, it is usually the practice nurse who monitors the blood of patients on DMARDs, or administers their injections. These encounters are an excellent opportunity to gain information about their condition and assess the patients' knowledge of their therapy. However, to provide high-quality care to all those who need it, community nurses need in-depth knowledge of the rheumatic diseases and their treatments. They also need a good working knowledge of the skills of other health professionals so that they can make swift and appropriate referrals.

Perhaps the most effective care is the 'shared-care' option, where the patient is managed within the primary sector, and specialist knowledge is sought from the secondary sector. This form of care requires close cooperation, active communication and the development of common systems. Community nurses and clinical nurse specialists (CNS) are often the link persons within the team who liaise and ensure a seamless service. The CNS is an excellent source of knowledge who can be relied upon to advise and support other nurses and patients in the primary sector.

Wherever and by whomsoever the patient is cared for, it should be remembered that patient education is the foundation of the most effective patient care. Treating the patients' symptoms will help them in the short term, teaching them will help them throughout their lives.

Useful Addresses

The addresses given below include those useful to community nurses wanting more information about professional matters, as well as patient support groups and organizations. Nurses working in general practice will encounter patients with rarer rheumatic disease not discussed in this handbook. Useful addresses for these diseases are also given.

Arthritis Care
8 Stephenson Way
London NW1 2HD
Tel: 0171 916 1500
Helpline: 0800 289170

The Arthritis Research Campaign (ARC)
Copemen House
St Mary's Court
St Mary's Gate
Chesterfield
Derbyshire S41 7TD
Tel: 01246 558033

British Acupuncture Council
Park House
206–208 Latimer Road
London W10 6RE
Tel: 020 8964 0222

British Association for Counselling (BAC)
1 Regent Place
Rugby
Warwickshire CV21 2PJ
Tel: 01788 578328

British Complementary Medicine Association (BCMA)
St Charles Hospital
Exmoor Street
London W10 6DZ
Tel: 020 8964 1205

British Council of Organisations of Disabled People (BCODP)
Litchurch Plaza
Litchurch Lane
Derby DE24 8AA
Tel: 01332 295551

British Health Professionals in Rheumatology (BHPR)
41 Eagle Street
London WC1R 4AR
Tel: 020 7242 3313

British League Against Rheumatism (BLAR)
41 Eagle Street
London WC1R 4AR
Tel: 020 7242 3313

British Sjögren's Syndrome Association
20 Kingstone Way
Nailsea
Bristol BS19 2RA
Tel: 01275 854215

British Society for Rheumatology (BSR)
41 Eagle Street
London WC1R 4AR
Tel: 020 7242 3313

Carers National Association
Ruth Pitter House
20–25 Glasshouse Yard
London EC1A 4JS
Tel: 020 7490 8818

Children's Chronic Arthritis Association
47 Battenhall Avenue
Worcester WR5 2HN
Tel: 01905 763556

Disabled Living Foundation
380–384 Harrow Road
London W14 3NS
Tel: 020 7289 6111

Ehlers-Danlos Support Group
Valerie Burrows Founder/Organizer
1 Chandler Close
Richmond
North Yorkshire DL10 5QQ
Tel: 01748 823867

Fibromyalgia Support Group
PO Box 206
Stourbridge DY9 8YL

Lupus UK
Queens Court
1 Eastern Road
Romford
Essex RM1 3NH
Tel: 01708 731251

Motability
Goodman House
Station Approach
Harlow
Essex CM20 2ET
Tel: 01279 635999

National Ankylosing Spondylitis Society (NASS)
3 Grosvenor Crescent
London SWX 7ER
Tel: 020 7235 9585

National Back Pain Association
16 Elm Tree Road
Teddington
Middlesex TW11 8ST
Tel: 020 8977 5474

Raynaud's and Scleroderma Association
112 Crewe Road
Alsager
Cheshire ST7 2JA
Tel: 01270 872776

Psoriatic Arthropathy Alliance
PO Box 111
St Albans
Hertfordshire AL2 3JQ
Tel: 01923 672837

National Association to Aid the Sexual and Personal Relationships
of People with Disability (SPOD)
286 Camden Road
London NW7 0BJ
Tel: 020 76078851

National Osteoporosis Society
PO Box 10
Radstock
Bath BA3 3YB
Tel: 01761 471771
Helpline: 01761 472721

RCN Rheumatology Nursing Forum
20 Cavendish Square
London W1M 0AB
Tel: 020 7409 3333

References

Affleck G, Fifield J, Pfeiffer C, Tennen H (1988) Social support and psychological adjustment to rheumatoid arthritis. Arthritis Care and Research 1: 71–77.

Aho K, Koskenvuom M, Tuominen J, Kaprio J (1986) Occurrence of rheumatoid arthritis in a nationwide series of twins. Journal of Rheumatology 13: 899–902.

Akil M, Amos RS, Steward P (1996) Infertility may sometimes be associated with NSAID consumption. British Journal of Rheumatology 35(1): 76–78.

Amos R, Pullar T, Capell H et al. (1986) Sulphasalazine for rheumatoid arthritis toxicity in 774 patients monitored for 1–11 years. British Medical Journal 293: 420–423.

Arnett FC, Edworthy SM, Bloch DA, McShane DJ, Fries JF, Cooper NS, Healey LA, Kaplan SR, Liang MH, Luthra HS, Medsger Jnr TA, Mitchell DM, Neustadt DH, Pinals RS, Schaller JG, Sharp JT, Wilder RL, Hunder GG (1988) The American Rheumatism Association 1987 Revised Criteria for the Classification of Rheumatoid Arthritis. Arthritis and Rheumatism 31: 315–324.

Arthritis Care (1994) Community Health Care for People with Arthritis. Quality Guidelines No 3. London: Arthritis Care.

Arthur V (1998) The rheumatic conditions: an overview. In: Hill J (Ed) Rheumatology Nursing: A Creative Approach. Edinburgh: Churchill Livingstone.

Aubin M, Marks R (1995) The efficacy of short-term treatment with transcutaneous electrical nerve stimulation for osteoarthritis knee pain. Physiotherapy 81(11): 669–675.

Bailey JJ, Black ME, Wilkin D (1994) Specialist outreach clinics in general practice. British Medical Journal 308: 1083–1086.

Bandura A (1977) Self-efficacy: towards a unifying theory of behavioural change. Psychological Review 84: 191–215.

Barlow DH (1994) Advisory Group on Osteoporosis Report. London: Department of Health.

Barlow JH, Williams B, Wright C (1996) Community based arthritis self management courses for older people. British Journal of Rheumatology 35(Abstract Suppl. 2 no. 52): 31.

Barrett CW, Tones J (1992) Shared care: the way forward. Hospital Update Plus 18: 7–10.

Bennet RM, Clark SR, Campbell SM, Burckhardt CS (1992) Low levels of somatomedin C in patients with fibromyalgia syndrome. Arthritis and Rheumatism 35 (10): 1113–1116.

Bird W (1993) Treatment in steps relieves the pain of osteoarthritis. Mims Magazine Weekly 22 June, 20–30.

Bird W (1994) Rheumatological audit – a general practice perspective. European Journal of Rheumatology 14 (Suppl.) issue 3: 3–4.

Bishop GP, Caro X, Fletcher EM, Russel IJ, Wolfe F (1990) Health locus of control and clinical outcome with fibrositis. Unpublished manuscript, University of Texas, San Antonio.

Blaaw A, Schuwith I, Van der Vleuten C, Smitz F, Van der Linden S (1995) Assessing clinical competence: recognition of case descriptions of rheumatic diseases by general practitioners. British Journal of Rheumatology 34: 375–379.

Blake D, Richard M, Graciela S, Alarcon HL, Brown SM (1987) Sexual quality of life: patients with arthritis compared to arthritis free controls. Journal of Rheumatology 14: 570–576.

Blaxter M (1990) Health and Lifestyles. London: Tavistock, Routledge.

Brennen P, Silman A J (1994) Breastfeeding and the onset of rheumatoid arthritis. Arthritis and Rheumatism 37: 808–813.

British League Against Rheumatism (1997) Standards of care for osteoarthritis (OA) and rheumatoid arthritis. London: BLAR.

British Society for Rheumatology (1992) Guidelines and audit measures for the specialist supervision of patients with rheumatoid arthritis. Journal of the Royal College of Physicians 26: 76–82.

Bunning RD, Materson RS (1991) A rational program of exercise for patients with osteoarthritis. Seminars in Arthritis and Rheumatism 21 (Suppl. 2): 33–43.

Burckhardt CS, Mannerkorphi K, Hedenberg L, Bjelle A (1994) A randomised controlled clinical trial of education and physical training for women with fibromyalgia. Journal of Rheumatology 21 (4): 714–720.

Callahan L, Brooks RH, Pincus T (1988) Further analysis of learned helplessness in rheumatological arthritis. Using a rheumatology attitude index. Journal of Rheumatology 15(3): 418–426.

Campbell BF, Sengupta S, Santos C, Lorig KR (1995) Balanced incomplete block design: descriptions, case study, and implications for practice. Health Education Quarterly 22: 201–210.

Carnell J (1998) Real lives, real solutions. Nursing Times 94 (42): 60–61.

Cawthorn A, Billingham J (1998) Complementary therapeutic intervention. In: Hill J (Ed) Rheumatology Nursing: A Creative Approach. Edinburgh: Churchill Livingstone.

Chapuy MC, Arlot ME, Duboenf FA, Brun J, Crouzet B, Arnaud S, Delmus P D, Meunier PJ (1992) Vitamin D3 and calcium to prevent hip fracture in elderly women. New England Journal of Medicine 327: 1637–1642.

Charlton C, Fleming D, McCormick A (1995) Morbidity Statistics from General Practice. London: HMSO.

Choy EHS, Kingsley G, Corkhill MM, Panayi GS (1993) Intramuscular methylprednisolone is superior to pulse oral methylprednisolone during the induction phase of chrysotherapy. British Journal of Rheumatology 32: 734–739.

Christiansen C, Krane S (1993) Advances in Corticosteroids. A Seminar in Print. USA: Adis International Inc.

Christiansen C, Riis BJ, Rodbro PC (1987) Prediction of rapid bone loss in post-menopausal women. Lancet 1: 1105–1108.

Cleland LG, James MJ (1997) Rheumatoid arthritis and the balance of n-6 n-3 essential fatty acids. British Journal of Rheumatology 36: 513–515.

Cohen ML (1994) Principles of pain and pain management. In: Klippel J, Dieppe P (Eds) Rheumatology. London: Mosby Year Book.

Compston JE, Rosen CJ (1997) Fast Facts: Osteoporosis. Oxford: Health Press.

Cooper C (1993) Epidemiology and public health impact of osteoporosis In: Reid DM (Ed) Osteoporosis. Baillière's Clinical Rheumatology 7(3): 459–477.

Cooper C (1995) Occupational activity and the risk of osteoarthritis. Journal of Rheumatology 22: (Suppl. 43) 10–12.

Cooper C (1998) Osteoarthritis epidemiology. In: Klippel JH, Dieppe PA (Eds) Rheumatology, 2nd edn. St Louis, MO: Mosby.

Cooper C, Atkinson EJ, O'Fallon WM, Melton LJ (1992) The incidence of clinically diagnosed vertebral fractures: a population based study in Rochester, Minnesota. Journal of Bone and Mineral Research 7: 221–227.

Cooper C, McAlindon T, Snow S (1994) Mechanical and constitutional factors for symptomatic knee osteoarthritis: differences between medial tibiofemoral and patellofemoral disease. Journal of Rheumatology 21: 307–313.

Creed F, Jason MV, Murphy S (1990) Measurement of psychiatric disorder in rheumatoid arthritis. Journal of Psychosomatic Research 34(1): 79–87.

Croft P, Coggan D, Cruddas M, Cooper C (1992) Osteoarthritis of the hip: an occupational disease in farmers. British Medical Journal 304: 1269–1272.

Dailey PA, Bishop GD, Russell IJ, Fletcher EM (1990) Psychological stress and the fibromyalgia syndrome. Journal of Rheumatology 17 (10): 1380–1385.

Dargie L, Proctor J (1993) Arthritis clinics in practice. Practice Nurse 1–14(6): 144–148.

Dargie L, Proctor J (1994) Setting up an arthritis clinic. Community Outlook 4 (7): 14–17.

Dargie L, Proctor J (1998) Seamless care. In: Hill J (Ed) Rheumatology Nursing: A Creative Approach. Edinburgh: Churchill Livingstone.

Darlington LG, Ramsay NW, Mansfield JR (1986) Placebo controlled, blind study of dietary manipulation therapy in rheumatoid arthritis. Lancet 1: 236–238.

Davis MS, Ettinger WH, Neuhaus JM, Mallon KP (1991) Knee osteoarthritis and physical functioning: evidence from the NHANES–1. Epidemiologic follow-up survey. Journal of Rheumatology 18: 591–598.

Day R (1994) Pharmacologic approaches, SAARD 1. In: Klippel J, Dieppe P (Eds) Rheumatology. London: Mosby Year Book.

Department of Health (1989) The NHS and Community Care Act. London: HMSO.

Department of Health (1998) The New NHS: Modern, Dependable. London: HMSO.

DeVellis BM (1993) Depression in rheumatological diseases. In: Newman S, Shipley M (Eds) Psychological Aspects in Rheumatic Disease. Baillière's Clinical Rheumatology 7(2): 241–258.

DeVellis RF, Blalock SJ (1993) Psychological and Educational Interventions to Reduce Arthritis Disability. Baillière's Clinical Rheumatology 7: 397–416.

Devins GM, Eworthy SM, Kleen GM, Manden H, Paul LC, Sealand TP (1993) Differences in illness intrusiveness across rheumatoid arthritis, end stage renal disease and multiple sclerosis. Journal of Neurology and Mental Disorders 181: 377–381.

Dickson J (1993) GP's joint approach to rheumatoid arthritis. Mims Magazine Weekly 2 February: 24–35.

Dieppe PA (1995) Therapeutic targets in OA. In: Osteoarthritis – Challenges for the 21st Century. Journal of Rheumatology 22: (Suppl.) 43: 1–160.

Dixon R, Christy N (1980) On the various forms of corticosteroid withdrawal syndrome. American Journal of Medicine 68: 224–230.

Donnelly S, Scott DL, Emery P (1992) The long term outcome and justification for early treatment. Clinical Rheumatology 6 (2): 251–260.

Donovan JL, Blake D (1992) Patient compliance, deviance or reasoned decision making? Social Science and Medicine 34: 507–513.

Donovan JL, Blake DR, Fleming G (1989) The patient is not a blank sheet: lay beliefs and their relevance to patient education. British Journal of Rheumatology 28: 58–61.

Douglas J, Byrne J (1998) Skin and nutrition. In: Hill J (Ed) Rheumatology Nursing: A Creative Approach. Edinburgh: Churchill Livingstone.

Durelte MR, Rodriguez AA, Agre JC, Silverman JL (1991) Needle electromyographic evaluation of patients with myofascial or fibromyalgia pain. American Journal of Physical and Medical Rehabilitation 70(3): 154–156.

Felson DT, Zhang Y, Anthony JM, Naimark A, Anderson JJ (1992) Weight loss reduces the risk for symptomatic knee osteoarthritis in women: the Framingham study. Annals of Internal Medicine 116: 535–539.

Fitzpatrick R, Lamb R, Newman S, Shipley M (1988) Social relationships and psychological well being in rheumatoid arthritis. Arthritis Care and Research 4: 63–72.

Fries JF, Spitz P, Kraines RG, Holman H (1980) Measurement of patient outcome in arthritis. Arthritis and Rheumatism 23: 137–145.

Frymoyer JW, Cats-Baril WL (1991) An overview of the incidence and cost of low back pain. Orthopaedic Clinics of North America 22: 261–271.

Furst DE (1988) The basis for variability of response to anti rheumatic drugs. In: Brooks P (Ed) Anti Rheumatic Drugs. Baillières Clinical Rheumatology. London: Baillière Tindall.

Gallagher JC, Melton W, Riggs BL, Bergstralh E (1980) Epidemiology of fractures of the proximal femur in Rochester, Minnesota. Clinical Orthopaedics and Related Research 150: 163–171.

George E, Kirwan JR (1990) Corticosteroid therapy in RA. Baillières Clinical Rheumatology 4: 621–647.

Goldsmith NF, Johnston JO (1975) Bone mineral: effects of oral contraceptives, pregnancy and lactation. Journal of Bone Surgery 657–668.

Goodwin D (1994) The case for outreach care in general practice. Rheumatology in Practice 1: 18–20.

Goodwin JS, Regan M (1982) Cognitive dysfunction associated with naproxen and ibuprofen in the elderly. Arthritis and Rheumatism 25: 1013–1015.

Greenfield S, Fitzcharles MA, Esdaile JM (1992) Reactive fibromyalgia syndrome. Arthritis and Rheumatism 35(6): 678–681.

Hammond A (1994) Joint protection behaviour in patients with rheumatoid arthritis following an education program. Arthritis Care and Research 7: 5–9.

Hampson SE, Glasgow RE, Zeiss AM, Birskovich SF, Foster L, Lines A (1993) Self-management of osteoarthritis. Arthritis Care Research 6: 17–22.

Harper D C (1983) Personality concepts and degrees of impairment in male adolescents with progressive and non-progressive physical disabilities. Journal of Clinical Psychology 39 (6): 857–867.

Havelock M (1998) Audit of compliance of the monitoring of slow acting anti-rheumatic and cytotoxic agents in rheumatology out-patients. Presentation at the Royal College of Nursing Rheumatology Conference – Measuring Outcomes, Bath, 1995.

Helliwell P (1996) Comparison of a community clinic with a hospital outpatient clinic in rheumatology. British Journal of Rheumatology 35: 385–388.

Helliwell P, O'Hara M (1995) Shared care between hospital and general practice: an audit of disease-modifying anti-rheumatic drugs monitoring in rheumatoid arthritis. British Journal of Rheumatology 34: 673–676.

Henriksson CM (1994) Long-term effects of fibromyalgia on everyday life. A study of 56 patients. Scandanavian Journal of Rheumatology 23(1): 36–41.

Hickman M, Drummond N, Grimshaw J (1994) A taxonomy of shared care for chronic disease. Journal of Public Health Medicine 16(4): 447–454.

Hill J (1985) Nursing clinics for arthritis. Nursing Times 81: 33–34.

Hill J (1995) Patient education in rheumatic disease. Nursing Standard 9: 25–28

Hill J (1997a) A practical guide to patient education and information giving. In: Woolfe AD, Van Riel PLCM (Eds) Clinical Rheumatology – Early Rheumatoid Arthritis. London: Baillière Tindall.

Hill J (1997b) Editorial: The expanding role of the nurse in rheumatology. British Journal of Rheumatology 36: 410–412.

Hill J (1998a) Rheumatology Nursing: A Creative Approach. Edinburgh: Churchill Livingstone.

Hill J (1998b) Patient education. In: Hill J (Ed) Rheumatology Nursing: A Creative Approach. Edinburgh: Churchill Livingstone.

Hill J (1998c) Pain and stiffness. In: Hill J (Ed) Rheumatology Nursing: A Creative Approach. Edinburgh: Churchill Livingstone.

Hill J, Bird HA, Lawton CW, Wright V (1990) The Arthritis Impact Measurement Scales: an anglicised version to assess the outcome of British patients with rheumatoid arthritis. British Journal of Rheumatology 29: 193–196.

Hill J, Bird HA, Hopkins R, Lawton C, Wright V (1991) The development and use of a patient knowledge questionnaire in rheumatoid arthritis. British Journal of Rheumatology 30: 45–49.

Hill J, Bird HA, Harmer R, Wright V, Lawton C (1994) An evaluation of the effectiveness, safety and acceptability of a nurse practitioner in a rheumatology outpatient clinic. British Journal of Rheumatology 33: 283–288.

Hill J, Bird HA, Harmer R, Bradley M (1997) Do drug information leaflets increase knowledge and if so does verbal backup enhance the effects. Arthritis and Rheumatism 40 (Suppl): S272, 1445.

Hirano PC, Laurent DD, Lorig K (1994) Arthritis patient education studies, 1987–1991: a review of the literature. Patient Education and Counselling 24: 9–54.

Hirsch BJ, Reich T (1985) Social networks and developmental psychopathology. A comparison of adolescent children of a depressed, arthritic or normal parent. Journal of Abnormal Psychology 94: 272–281.

Huskisson EC, Woolf PC, Bourne HW, Scott J, Franklyn S (1974) Four anti inflammatory drugs – response and variations. British Medical Journal 1: 1084–1089.

Hyde V (1995) Community nursing: a unified discipline? In: Cain P, Hyde V, Hawkins E (Eds) Community Nursing: Dimensions and Dilemmas. London: Arnold.

Jamison RM (1996) Comprehensive pre-treatment and outcome assessment for chronic opioid therapy. Journal of Pain Symptom Management 11: 231–241.

Katz P, Yelin LH (1995) The development of depressive symptoms among women with rheumatoid arthritis. Arthritis and Rheumatism 38: 49–56.

Kay A (1986) European League Against Rheumatism study of adverse reactions to D-penicillamine. British Journal of Rheumatology 25: 193–198.

Kay A, Puller T (1992) Variations among rheumatologists in prescribing and monitoring of disease-modifying anti-rheumatic drugs. British Journal of Rheumatology 31: 477–483.

Kellgren JH, Moore R (1952) Generalized osteoarthritis and Heberden's nodes. British Journal of Medicine 1: 181–187.

Kirwan JR (1994) Systemic corticosteroids in rheumatology. In: Klippel JH, Dieppe P (Eds) Rheumatology. London: Mosby Year Book.

Kirwan JR (1995) The effects of glucocorticoid steroid on joint destruction in RA. New England Journal of Medicine 333: 142–146.

Kirwan JR (1996) Rheumatology outpatient workload increases inexorably. British Journal of Rheumatology 35 (Abstract Suppl. 2): no. 48.

Kirwan J, Reeback JS (1986) Stanford Health Assessment Questionnaire modified to access disability in British patients with rheumatoid arthritis. British Journal of Rheumatology 25: 206–209.

Kovar P, Allegrante JP, Mackenzie R, Peterson MGER, Gutin B, Charlson ME (1992) Supervised fitness walking in patients with osteoarthritis of the knee. Annals of Internal Medicine 121: 133–140.

Kremer JM, Joong KL (1986) The safety and efficacy of the use of methotrexate in long term therapy for rheumatoid arthritis. Arthritis and Rheumatism 29: 822–831.

Krueger DW (1984) Rehabilitation Psychology. Maryland, CO: Aspin.

Kumar VN, Redford GB (1982) Transcutaneous nerve stimulation in rheumatoid arthritis. Archives of Physical Medicine and Rehabilitation 63: 595–596.

Langer EJ (1983) The Psychology of Control. Thousand Oaks, CA: Sage.

Lawrence JS (1961) Prevalence of rheumatoid arthritis. Annals of the Rheumatic Diseases 20: 11–17.

Le Gallez P (1990) Osteoarthritis (2): Care of the patient. Practice Nurse 3: 176–177.

Le Gallez P (1993) Rheumatoid arthritis: effects on the family. Nursing Standard 7 (39): 30–34.

Le Gallez P (1995) Rheumatoid arthritis. Primary Health Care 5 (7): 449–462.

Le Gallez P (1998) Teratogenesis and drugs for rheumatic disease. Nursing Times 84(27): 41– 44.

Lehmann JF (1990) Therapeutic Heat and Cold, 4th edn. Baltimore: Williams & Wilkins.

Lentall G, Hetherington T, Egon M, Morgan M (1992) The use of thermal agents to influence the effectiveness of low-load prolonged stretch. Journal of Orthopaedic and Sport Physical Therapy 16(5): 200–201.

Leonard PA, Bienz SR, Clegg DD, Ward JR (1987) Haematuria in patients with rheumatoid arthritis receiving gold and penicillamine. Journal of Rheumatology 14: 55–59.

Lorig K (1996) Patient Education – A Practical Approach. Thousand Oaks, CA: Sage.

Lorig K, Lubeck D, Kraines RG, Seleznick M, Holman HR (1985) Outcomes of self-help education for patients with arthritis. Arthritis and Rheumatism 28: 680–685.

Lorig K, Chastain R, Holman H, Lubeck D, Seleznick M, Ung E (1989) The beneficial outcome of the arthritis self management course are not adequately explained by behavioural change. Arthritis and Rheumatism 32: 91–95.

MacGregor AJ, Silman AJ (1998) Rheumatoid arthritis – classification and epidemiology. In: Klippel JH, Dieppe PA (Eds) Rheumatology, 2nd edn. London: Mosby.

Manne SL, Zautra AJ (1989) Spouse criticism and support: their association with coping and psychological adjustment among people with rheumatoid arthritis. Journal of Personal Social Psychology 56: 608–617.

Marks R, Quinney AH, Wessel J (1993) Reliability and validity of the measurement of position sense in women with osteoarthritis of the knee. Journal of Rheumatology 20: 1919–1924.

Martin J, Meltzer H, Elliot D (1988) The prevalence of disability among adults. OPCS surveys of disability in Great Britain. Report 1, OPCS Social Surveys Division. London: HMSO.

Matthew A, Humphreys CA (1994) Rheumatoid arthritis. In: Davis PS (Ed) Nursing the Orthopaedic Patient. Edinburgh: Churchill Livingstone.

Maycock J (1988) The image of rheumatic disease. In: Salter M (Ed) Altered Body Image: The Nurse's Role. New York: Wiley .

McAlindon T, Felson DT (1997) Nutrition: risk factors for osteoarthritis. Annals of the Rheumatic Diseases 56: 397–402.

Meenan RF, Gertman PM, Mason JH (1980) Measuring health status in arthritis: the Arthritis Impact Measurement Scales. Arthritis and Rheumatism 23 (2): 146–152.

Melton LJ III (1988) Epidemiology of fractures. In: Riggs BL, Melton LJ III (Eds) Etiology, Diagnosis and Management. New York: Raven Press.

Miller JF (1992) Coping with Chronic Illness, Overcoming Powerlessness, 2nd edn. London: FA Davies.

Minor MA (1994) Exercise in the management of osteoarthritis of the knee and hip. Arthritis Care Research 7: 198–204.

Moldofsky HP, Chester WJ (1970) Pain and mood pattern in patients with rheumatoid arthritis. A prospective study. Psychosomatic Medicare 32: 309–318.

Mooney J (1996) Audit of a rheumatology nurse outreach clinic. Rheumatology in Practice (Winter): 18–20.

Newman SP (1993) Coping with rheumatoid arthritis. Annals of the Rheumatic Diseases 52: 553–554.

Nicassio PM, Wallston KA (1992) Longitudinal relationships among pain, sleep problems and depression in rheumatoid arthritis. Journal of Abnormal Psychology 101 (3): 514–520.

Nienhuis R, Hoekstra A (1984) Transcutaneous electronic nerve stimulation in ankylosing spondylitis. Arthritis and Rheumatism 27: 1074–1075.

Nilsson BE, Westlin NE (1971) Bone density in athletes. Clinical Orthopaedics 77: 179–182.

Nordenskiold V (1994) Evaluation of assistive devices after a course in joint protection. International Journal of Technology Assessment in Health Care 10: 293–304.

Oliveria SA, Felson DT, Reed JI, Cirillo PA, Walker AM (1995) Incidence of symptomatic hand, hip and knee osteoarthritis among patients in a health maintenance organisation. Arthritis and Rheumatism 38: 1134–1141.

OPCS (1989) General Household Survey. London: HMSO.

Parker JC, Wright GE (1995) The implications of depression for pain and disability in rheumatoid arthritis. Arthritis Care and Research 8(4): 279–283.

Pattison D (1998) Fed-up with nutrition. Journal of Orthopaedic Nursing 2: 105–115.

Phelan MJ, Byrne J, Campbell A, Lynch M (1992) A profile of rheumatology nurse specialists in the United Kingdom (letter). British Journal of Rheumatology 31 (2): 858.

Phelan M, Campbell A, Byrne J, Hough Y, Hunt J, Lynch M (1994) The effects of an education programme on the perceptions of arthritis by spouses of patients with rheumatoid arthritis. Scandinavian Journal of Rheumatology (Suppl. 74).

Pigg JS, Caniff R, Driscoll PW (1985) Rheumatology Nursing. A Problem Orientated Approach. New York: Wiley.

Pocock NA, Eisman HA, Yeates MG, Sambrook PN, Eberl S (1986) Physical activity is a determinant of femoral neck and lumbar spine density. Journal of Clinical Investigation 78: 618–621.

Prady J, Vale A, Hill J (1998) Body image and sexuality. In: Hill J (Ed) Rheumatology Nursing: A Creative Approach. Edinburgh: Churchill Livingstone.

Radojenic V, Nicassio PM, Weisman MH (1992) Behaviour intervention with and without family support for rheumatoid arthritis. Behavioural Therapy 23: 13–30.

Recker RR, Karpf DB, Quan H et al. (1995) Three Year Treatment of Osteoporosis with Alendronate: Effects on Vertebral Fracture Incidence. Abstracts of the 77th Annual Meeting of the Endocrine Society, Washington DC.

Reif L (1975) Beyond medical interventions: strategies for managing life in the face of chronic illness. In: Davies M, Kramer M, Straws A (Eds) Nurses in Practice: A Perspective on Work Environments. St Louis, MO: Mosby.

Reisine S (1993) Marital status and social support in rheumatoid arthritis. Arthritis and Rheumatism 36: 589–592 .

Reisine S (1995) Arthritis and the family. Arthritis Care and Research 8 (4): 265–271.

Reisine S, Goodenow C, Grady KE (1987) The impact of rheumatoid arthritis on the home maker. Social Science and Medicine 25: 89–95.

Revenson TA, Majerovitz DM (1991) The effects of illness on the spouse, social resources as stress buffers. Arthritis Care and Research 4: 63–72.

Richardson A (1992) Rheumatoid arthritis in pregnancy. Nursing Standard 6(45): 25–29.

Ritchie DM, Boyle JA, McInnes JM, Jasani MK, Dalakos TG, Grieveson P, Buchanan WW (1968) Studies with an articular index for assessment of joint tenderness in patients with rheumatoid arthritis. Quarterly Journal of Medicine 147: 393–406.

Rook K (1990) Social networks as a source of social control in older adult lines. In: Giles H, Coupeland N, Weimann J M (Eds) Communication Health and The Elderly. Manchester: University of Manchester.

Rotter JB (1966) Generalised expectations for internal versus external control of reinforcement. Psychological Monographs 80 (1): 1–28.

Ryan S (1995a) Sharing care in an out-patients' clinic. Nursing Standard 10: 23–25.

Ryan S (1995b) Fibromyalgia: what help can nurses give? Nursing Standard 9: 25–28.

Ryan S (1995c) Nutrition and the rheumatoid patient. British Journal of Nursing 4(3): 132–136.

Ryan S (1996) Does inflammatory arthritis affect sexuality? British Journal of Rheumatology 35 (Supplement): 19.

Shaul M (1995) From early twinges in mastery, the process of adjustment in living with rheumatoid arthritis. Arthritis Care and Research 8(4): 290–297.

Silman AJ, Davies P, Curry HLF, Evans SJW (1983) Is rheumatoid arthritis becoming less severe? Journal of Chronic Diseases 36: 891–897.

Silman AJ, Kay A, Brennan P (1992) Timing of pregnancy in relation to the onset of rheumatoid arthritis. Arthritis Rheumatism 35: 152–155.

Silman AJ, MacGregor AJ, Thomson W, Holligan S, Carthy D, Farhan A, Ollier WER (1993) Twin concordance rates for rheumatoid arthritis: results from a nationwide study. British Journal of Rheumatology 32: 903–907.

Slemenda CW, Christian JC, Williams CJ, Norton JA, Johnston CC Jr. (1991) Genetic determinants of bone mass in adult women: a re-evaluation of the twin model and the potential importance of gene interaction on heritability estimates. Journal of Bone Mineral Research 6: 561–567.

Smruti Riley H (1998) Role of the physiotherapist in rheumatology. In: Le Gallez P (Ed) Rheumatology for Nurses: Patient Care. London: Whurr Publishers.

Snaith M (1994) Outreach specialist rheumatology clinics in a primary care setting. Journal of Primary Care Rheumatology 1: 4–5.

Snaith ML (1996) ABC of Rheumatology. London: BMJ Publishing Group.

Spector TD, Hochberg MC (1990) The protective effect of the oral contraceptive pill on rheumatoid arthritis. An overview of the analytical epidemiological studies using meta-analysis. Journal of Clinical Epidemiology 43: 1121–1130.

Spector TD, Hard DJ, Powell RJ (1993) Prevalence of rheumatoid factor in women: evidence for a secular decline. Annals of Rheumatic Disease 52: 254–257.

Stamp J (1998) The team approach to mobility and self care. In: Hill J (Ed) Rheumatology Nursing: A Creative Approach. Edinburgh: Churchill Livingstone.

Storm T, Thamsborg G, Steiniche T, Genant H, Sorenson OH (1990) Effects of intermittent cyclical etidronate therapy on bone mass and fracture rate in women with postmenopausal osteoporosis. New England Journal of Medicine 322: 1265–1271.

Strenstrom CH (1994) Therapeutic exercise in rheumatoid arthritis. Arthritis Care Research 7: 190–197

Sturdy C (1998a) Surgical interventions. In: Hill J (Ed) Rheumatology Nursing: A Creative Approach. Edinburgh: Churchill Livingstone.

Sturdy C (1998b) Assessing rheumatic patients. In: Hill J (Ed) Rheumatology Nursing: A Creative Approach. Edinburgh: Churchill Livingstone.

Summers MN, Haley WE, Reveille JO, Alarcon GS (1988) Radiographic assessment and psychological variables as predictors of pain and functional impairment in osteoarthritis of the knee or hip. Arthritis and Rheumatism 31: 204–209.

Symmons DPM, Barrett EM, Bankhead CR, Scott, DGI, Silman AJ (1994) The incidence of rheumatoid arthritis in the United Kingdom: results from the Norfolk Arthritis Register. British Journal of Rheumatology 33: 735–739.

Symmons D, Bankhead C (1994) Health care needs assessment for musculoskeletal disease: the first step estimating the number of incidents and prevalent cases. Chesterfield: Arthritis and Rheumatism Council for Research.

Thompson P, Dunne C (1995) NSAIDs Use and Abuse. Collected Reports on Rheumatic Diseases. Chesterfield: Arthritis and Rheumatism Council.

UKCC (1989) Exercising Accountability. London: UKCC.

UKCC (1992a) Scope of Professional Practice. London: UKCC.

UKCC (1992b) Code of Professional Conduct. London: UKCC.

UKCC (1992c) Standards for the Administration of Medicines. London: UKCC.

Van der Laar MAFJ, Van der Korst JK (1991) Rheumatoid arthritis, food and allergy. Seminars in Arthritis and Rheumatism 21: 12–23.

Vandenbrouke JP, Valkenburg HA, Boersma JW, Festen JJM, Cats A (1982) Oral contraceptives and rheumatoid arthritis: further evidence for a preventive effect. Lancet ii: 830–842.

Voyce MA (1998) Osteoporosis: its significance in rheumatoid disease. In: Le Gallez P (Ed) Rheumatology for Nurses: Patient Care. London: Whurr Publishers.

Walker D (1994) Outreach clinics – a consultant replies. Rheumatology in Practice 1: 6–8.

Wallston K (1993) Psychological control and its impact on the management of rheumatoid disorders. In: Newman S, Shipley M (Eds) Psychological Aspects of Rheumatic Disease. London: Baillière Tindall.

Weusten BLAM, Jacobs JWG, Bijlsma JWJ (1993) Corticosteroid pulse therapy in active RA. Seminars in Arthritis and Rheumatism 23: 183–192.

Widdows C (1998) The role of the podiatrist in rheumatology. In: Le Gallez P (Ed) Rheumatology for Nurses: Patient Care. London: Whurr Publishers.

Willis J (1998) The changing face of primary care across the UK. Nursing Times 94(12): 58–59.

Wilson Barnett J (1984) Key functions in nursing: the fourth Winifred Rapteal Memorial Lecture. London: Royal College of Nursing.

Wolfe F (1990) The American College of Rheumatology Criteria for the Classification of Fibromyalgia. Arthritis and Rheumatism 33(2): 160–172.

Wolfe F, Ross K, Anderson J, Russel W, Herbert L (1995) The prevalence and characteristics of fibromyalgia in the general population. Arthritis and Rheumatism 38: 19–28.

Yelin E, Callahan L (1995) The economic cost and social and psychological impact of musculo-skeletal conditions. Arthritis and Rheumatism 38: 1351–1362.

Yelin E, Henke C, Epstein W (1987) Work dynamics of the person with rheumatoid arthritis. Arthritis and Rheumatism 30: 507–512.

Zigmond AS, Snaith RP (1983) The Hospital Anxiety and Depression Scale. Acta Psychiatrica Scandinavica 67: 361–370.

Index

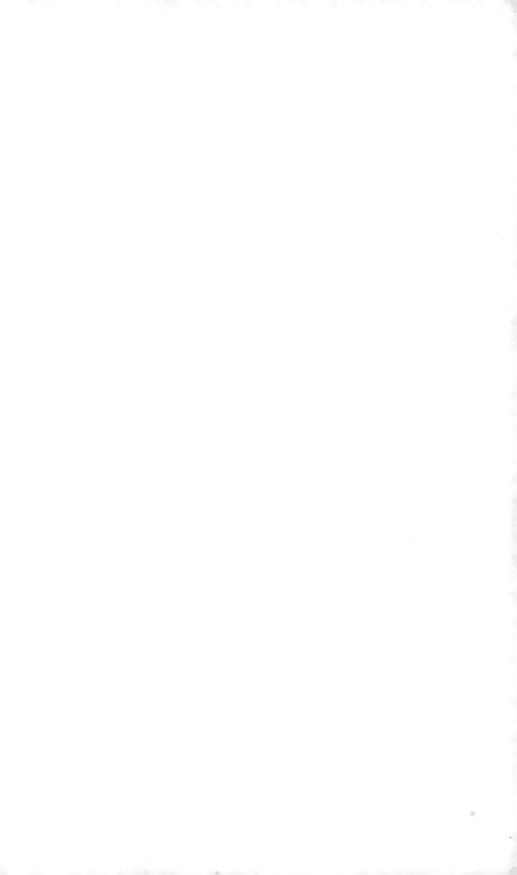